CONQUER HEADACHES

*How to get rid of
your headaches and
on with your life*

By Robert G. Ford, M.D.
Director, Ford Headache Clinic

and

Kay T. Ford, R.N.
Administrator, Ford Headache Clinic

THE EXPERTS SPEAK OUT...

"**O**nly occasionally does one see a medical book aimed at the patient, which is able to condense, make understandable, and relay information in a caring and hopeful manner. Robert and Kay Ford have achieved that, however, in this small but masterful book. It is the common symptoms that cause patients to come to doctors, and it is the variability of those symptoms that often cause doctors to misdiagnose common illnesses. This book explains the variations in the presentation of headache, how they can be approached diagnostically and therapeutically, and how they can be managed including, to some degree, by life-style changes. In total, the message for the patient is one of both understanding and hope: clearly an achievement to be appreciated in a medical book directed at patients.*

Further, this book, because it deals with an extremely common symptom, is also of great interest to practicing general physicians. It should aid them in understanding the problem of headaches so as to more effectively treat them. I believe, therefore, that this book, although directed at patients, will find great utility in the library of general physicians, as it unquestionably gives differential diagnoses and insights so important in everyday practice.

J. Claude Bennett, M.D.
President
The University of Alabama at Birmingham

"Conquer Your Headaches is easy to read, and I believe patients will like it...Two of the secretaries who work with me liked it very much, and it was reassuring to them that recurring headaches can be managed successfully."

Jack P. Whisnant, M.D.
President of the American Academy of Neurology
Mayo Clinic
Rochester, Minnesota
International authority on stroke

Conquer Your Headaches:
How to get rid of your headaches and on with your life
Published by International Headache Management, Inc.

Printing History
First edition published March 1994

ISBN 0-9636292-5-5

Published in the United States of America

Printed in the United States of America

PICTURE THIS SCENE...

•••

You are the youngest member of your family, a mere adolescent. For years, you have tended your father's sheep ranch. One day you are asked to deliver food to your brothers, soldiers in the King's army. When you arrive, you see a nine foot tall champion named Goliath, challenging the King's soldiers to a fight. For 40 days, Goliath has laughed at your brothers, and they are terrified, deadly afraid to face the giant who has incapacitated them, and who threatens to conquer them.

You go to the King. "I'll face Goliath," you tell him. You are his only volunteer. So the King dresses you in his own coat of armor, a bulky tunic and helmet and a large sword that drags the ground. But you take off the cumbersome armor, skip to the nearest creek, and gather some stones. Then, with sling in hand, you head off to challenge the mighty Goliath.

Goliath stands before you. He is huge and frightening. He wears a coat of heavy bronze armor, shin guards, and helmet. A spear and javelin hang over his back. With a bare back and a simple sling, you stand up to Goliath. You show no fear. You speak directly to him, and your words make him angry.

"You come against me with sword and spear and javelin, but I come against you in the name of the Lord Almighty, the God of the armies of Israel...."

You know the rest of the story. The shepherd boy, David, bravely swings his sling. The stone hits Goliath on the forehead and immediately kills him. David conquers the giant that no one else will dare face.

Life can present us with some Goliaths of our own. Sometimes these giants seem so titanic, they incapacitate us and threaten to destroy us. They can be huge and frightening. We are afraid to face them so we suffer with fear and pain.

Headaches are like giants. They interfere with our life, our work, our relationships, our joy. They intimidate and torment us. They threaten to overpower us. *Yet*, now there is hope for the one who suffers from the giant. New research, new medication, and dedicated physicians are your sling and stone. Headache can be conquered. Just as David stood up to Goliath, now is the time to face the headache that threatens to defeat you. Now is the time to conquer Goliath.

I Samuel 17:1-54

Cover: David—sculptured in marble in 1504 A.D. by Michelangelo—is displayed in Florence, Italy.

DEDICATED TO...

··

Janyce H. Townley and the memory of
Mary E. Ford—our mothers.

ACKNOWLEDGEMENTS

First of all, a loving thank you to William, our eleven-year-old, who exhibited patience far beyond his years while his parents were involved in writing and organizing this book. William, thanks so much for your understanding and cooperation, without which this book would not have been possible.

The authors also want to thank Denise George for her support, her many suggestions, and for providing us with the cover story on Michelangelo's David. To David Wimbish and KroutDavis Marketing, thank you for your assistance with preparation of the manuscript. And, Patrick Netter and Toni Boyle, thank you for ideas and your help in organizing the material.

A sincere thank you is also due the staff of the Ford Headache Clinic for their commitment to our patients, and their continuing efforts in the fight against head pain. We also want to express our thanks and appreciation to our colleagues throughout the world who are with us in this fight, and from whom we have learned much. And, finally, we also want to acknowledge and salute those men and women in the laboratories, the scientists whose breakthroughs in research have enabled us to gain the upper hand in the battle against our ancient enemy—the headache.

TABLE OF CONTENTS

. . . .

Part Three (Continued)

Part Four
The Prevention And Treatment
Of Headaches

Part Four (Continued)

TABLE OF CONTENTS

INDEX

···

I

Index A: *(Continued)*

Index B:
Illustrations

FOREWORD

∙∙∙

Bob and Kay Ford's book, *Conquer Your Headaches*, for the patient with headaches is simple yet comprehensive and unpretentious yet profound. It may become a best-seller. One cannot write authoritatively on headaches unless one is at least 55 years old, has evaluated and treated hundreds (perhaps thousands) of patients with headaches, has experienced headache himself (or herself), has read what others have written on the subject, has tried what others have tried, and has the philosophical outlook to accept small gains and an imperfect world. By these criteria, Robert Ford qualifies. This book is not about controlled clinical trials or brain peptide research, but about approaches which the authors find helpful to patients. As the title suggests, the authors are convinced that the patient can herself (himself) do something about headaches. Certain influences which trigger headaches can be avoided. There now are preventative medications and other medications for headaches. The authors also encourage a mind set and prayer. The authors provide a broad range of medications and injections to influence the pain experience.

A former professor of mine, Irwin Hilliard, claimed that medications were particularly helpful in relief of suffering if physicians believed in them. Robert and Kay Ford believe in the approaches they recommend, and I believe they can help patients with headaches.

Peter James Dyck, M.D.
Professor of Neurology
Mayo Medical School
Mayo Clinic
Rochester, Minnesota
Immediate Past President of the
American Neurological Association
International authority on neuropathy

FOREWORD

PREFACE

∙∙

This book was written for the millions of headache sufferers who struggle to survive under the burden and "thorn in the flesh" of headaches. Some who will read this are virtually incapacitated with recurrent headache—headache which interferes with family, employment, happiness, and general well-being. Others of you may have only an occasional headache, but you too, will find the information contained within these pages to be helpful. Here, we have attempted to answer most questions about headaches that have been asked by our patients.

Many of those who come to our clinic for help already have been to five or six doctors, including internists, general medical physicians, chiropractic physicians, oral and dental surgeons, ENT specialists, allergists, neurosurgeons, neurologists and psychiatrists—often without positive results. For this reason they arrive at our clinic skeptical, disillusioned, and sometimes having gone through several surgical procedures for headache without significant improvement. We often see patients who have taken pain medication on a daily basis for weeks, months, and sometimes for more than 30 years. They are worn out, depressed, sometimes on the verge of loss of job, and often they tell us that, "you are my last hope."

They want to find out why they suffer from headaches, why they feel so wretched day after day, why they awaken each morning facing another day of survival on over-the-counter or prescription medication to ward off the inevitable daily headache. For many of these people, if headache isn't present on awakening, it's there by mid-morning. There just doesn't seem to be any escape.

They ask questions such as, "What can be done?" "Is there any hope?" "Is my poor sleep pattern a result of, or part of, the actual headache, or is this some basic psychological problem?" Our patients tell us that other doctors told them the problem was just stress. Then they ask, "But why would stress wake me up from a sound sleep?" Other sufferers have been told their headaches are caused by depression—but is depression causing the headache, or is it the other way around? Patients ask us why they have continuous headaches seemingly in their sinus cavities, when their ear-nose-and-throat specialist found their sinuses to be clear. After visiting our clinic one of our patients said, "There are a lot of people walking around who think they have sinus problems, when in reality they have a migraine."

And, of course, questions about migraine are uppermost on the minds of many of our patients. They ask us about the cause or cure of migraine. They want to know why the nausea and vomiting associated with migraine can be so severe when no identifiable cause is present, and extensive testing for tumor, infection or bleeding has turned up nothing. Why do the strongest pain medications not provide more relief? Why do migraine attacks occur when they do?

Our patients want to know what role hormones, pregnancy, allergy, depression, and diet play in the formation of headaches. They want to be able to recognize the triggers that can bring on a headache. Many have noticed that changes in the weather seem to bring on a headache. Is this a recognized medical fact? Many want to cut back on the amount of pain medication they are taking.

Our patients want someone to believe in them, listen to them, and assure them that they are not really hypochondriacs. Of course, they want help on the basis of the latest medical knowledge. They want to know if there are ways to control headache other than with oral and injectable pain medications such as analgesics and prescription narcotics. They want to know that something is really wrong when so many tests, including CT scans, MRI scans, EEGs, X-rays, and so on, have been normal. Unfortunately, they have been told by other physicians many things including, "You'll just have to live with it." They may have been given the impression that the pain "doesn't really exist," that "it's all in your mind." And yet the pain is so real. It is certainly no "phantom," and there must be an alternative other than "learning to live with it." The headache patients want to know if physicians and their staffs truly know what they are going through.

We want this book to provide help to you as one of the millions who suffer from headaches. It is to you, the headache sufferer, that this book was written.

WHEN YOUR HEAD HURTS

• •

Had a headache lately?

Chances are that you have. In an average year, more than 90 per cent of the general population will suffer at least one headache—and most of us will have several.

For years, the headache has been the subject of teasing and laughter. Everyone knows the standard line: "Not tonight, dear. I have a headache!" And yet...a headache is certainly nothing to joke about. When your head hurts, the whole world can seem to be out of focus, and nothing is quite right.

There are many different types of headaches, with different causes—and, therefore, needing different treatments. But one thing to keep in mind is that there is almost always an effective treatment. [6, 7, 18, 19, 34, 38, 59, 61, 64, 65, 72, 73] No one should have to "put up" with a headache...no one should have to suffer in silence. That's why we have established the Ford Headache Clinic, and that's why we have prepared this book. Within the next few pages, we will discuss various types of headaches, including symptoms and treatments.

About 90 per cent of those who come to the Ford Headache Clinic either become headache free or see dramatic improvement in their condition. We may not be able to eliminate headaches altogether, but we're ready and anxious to take a giant step in that direction.

COMMON QUESTIONS ABOUT HEADACHES

· ·

How Common is Headache?
  No one knows exactly how many people in the United States suffer from chronic headaches—but there are millions of them. Estimates range from 30 million to 60 million. And remember that we're talking about those who regularly have to deal with head pain, and not just those who may occasionally have a headache.

  We do know that seventy-five percent of those who suffer from headaches are women. Figures (1) and (2) show the prevalence of migraine in men and women at about age forty, with women outnumbering men approximately three to one. In early childhood, girls and boys get headaches at about the same rate, with boys slightly outnumbering girls prior to puberty or menarche—but that changes with the onset of puberty. From that point on, females are three times more likely than men to suffer from chronic headaches. Roughly eight to ten per cent of all men and eighteen to twenty-five per cent of all women will suffer a migraine attack at some time.[36]

Where does headache pain come from?

  Just as there are many different types of headaches, there are many sources of headache pain. The source of your headache pain may be the brain itself, muscles of the face or head, and the brain coverings (meninges) or the blood vessels surrounding the brain. Pain may also come from the eyes and ears, teeth, jaws, and sinuses.[59] Headaches would be much easier to diagnose and treat if they were all the same, and if all patients responded the same way, but that just isn't the case.

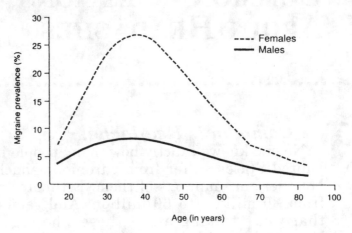

Figure 1. Migraine prevalence by age. Prevalence increased from 12 to 38 years of age in both females and males; the peak was considered higher among females. Used by permission from Richard B. Lipton, M.D., and Walter F. Stewart, Ph.D., M.P.H. (Supple. Ed.): Advances in biology and pharmacology of headache. Neurology Vol. 43, (6), Supplement 3, June, 1993.

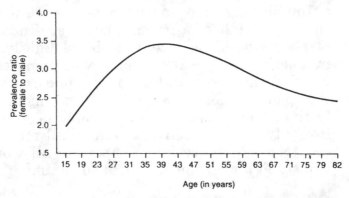

Figure 2. Prevalence ratio of female to male migraine sufferers by age. Ratio varied strikingly with age. Used by permission from Richard B. Lipton, M.D., and Walter F. Stewart, Ph.D., M.P.H. (Supple. Ed.): Advances in biology and pharmacology of headache. Neurology Vol. 43, (6), Supplement 3, June, 1993.

Do I have reason to be alarmed?

Most headaches are not symptoms of severe illness, nor are they life-threatening—although those good words may not help much when you feel like a band of Gremlins is playing The Anvil Chorus somewhere in your head. But even though most headaches are relatively harmless, a recurring headache should definitely be checked out by a doctor because it might mean there is another problem that needs attention. Some things to watch out for:

Sudden onset of an excruciatingly severe headache that is clearly different from headaches you've had previously.

A headache that seems to be steadily worsening instead of getting better.

A headache that is accompanied by disturbances of speech or vision; numbness, weakness or clumsiness of a limb; drowsiness, confusion, or memory loss.

Persistent headache following head injury.

Headache accompanied by other symptoms such as persistent fever, stiff neck, or persistent vomiting.

The appearance of severe headaches in anyone over 50 years of age. (Most "benign" types of headaches show up well before this age.)[59]

None of these symptoms is a sure sign that something serious is wrong with you—but they are reason enough to pay a visit to your doctor.

Are headaches really that "big of a deal?"

They certainly are. Beyond the plain truth that a headache hurts—they are also very costly. You can't watch more than a couple of hours of television without seeing at least one commercial for a headache remedy, and you'll probably see two or three of them. Headache treatment is big business for a number of American pharmaceutical companies...and no wonder: Every year, Americans spend more than $2.3 billion for over-the-counter pain remedies, mostly to rid themselves of headaches.

Add to that the cost of lost time from work, estimated cost of health care, and you'll come up with an average annual price tag in excess of $6 billion! It is also estimated that a whopping 155 million work days are lost each year because of headaches. If the American people were able to rid themselves of headaches once and for all, they would not only be healthier and thus, happier, but more prosperous to boot! [36]

Which pain-reliever should I buy?

Just about any over-the-counter headache medicine can give you temporary relief of pain, depending upon which is easiest on your system. The problem is that, for those who are chronic headache sufferers, none of the various headache medicines will do much good over the long-term. In fact, they may wind up doing more harm than good.

When any of these medicines are taken on a regular basis, the end result is what doctors refer to as "analgesic rebound headache." What happens is that these medications seem to change the way the brain works. Studies have shown that one-third of patients who take pain medication more than two days a week will actually have fewer headaches after being off the medicine for one month. After being off medication for three months, over 80 per cent will improve. [43, 44, 58]

What this means is that four out of five chronic headache sufferers who take excessive pain medication obtain significant relief, just by stopping their daily medication for three or four months. [36, 58, 72]

If you suffer from analgesic rebound headache, you may need to work with your doctor or headache specialist to get off pain medication. We will talk more about "analgesic rebound headache," in Part Three of this book.

At what age do headaches begin?

A person who is prone to headaches usually finds this out pretty early in life—and that's especially true of the person who is prone to migraines. The migraine headache usually makes its first appearance in a person's life during adolescence, and it is very rare for migraine to first show up after the age of 50. Childhood migraine may even affect children as young as three. Most of those who suffer with chronic headaches are women who have their first attacks around the onset of menstruation. At the same time, about 10 percent of women who suffer from migraine headaches say they first became afflicted after they turned 40—or right around the time of menopause. Only 3 to 5 per cent of migraine sufferers report having their first such headache after the age of 50. [61]

I get headaches during the middle of the night. Sometimes they wake me up out of a sound sleep. Should I be worried?

The person who is aroused out of a deep sleep by an intense headache may worry that something drastic is wrong. But that's usually not the case. Actually, it's fairly normal for a headache to attack its victim during the middle of the night —usually sometime between the hours of 2:00 and 5:00 a.m. This is especially true for those who have a tendency to suffer from migraine headaches. This person may be awakened not only by a throbbing headache, but by feelings of nausea or even vomiting.

The person who suffers from cluster headaches may experience attacks at the same time of the day or night on a regular basis. This type of headache may be related to a disturbance in the victim's wake-sleep cycle, so it's not at all uncommon for the headache to occur during the middle of the night. [34, 61]

We will talk more about migraine headaches in Part Two of this book, and we'll discuss cluster headaches in Part Three.

Of course, it's no fun at all to be awakened by a terrible headache. But there should be some relief, at least, in the knowledge that this is not necessarily a sign that something is seriously wrong.

THE MOTHER OF ALL HEADACHES: THE MIGRAINE

Why do we refer to migraine as "the mother" of all headaches?

Only those who have never experienced one would ask that question. A migraine headache is an intense, pounding pain in the head that can last for hours, or even days. In comparison, it can make a root canal seem like a day at the beach.

What follows are some of the most commonly asked questions about migraine headaches.

What is the difference between a migraine and an "ordinary" headache?

A migraine headache has at least four distinguishing characteristics:

1) Its intensity. A migraine headache is usually so intense that it may be referred to as a "sick headache," and may be accompanied by nausea and vomiting.

2) Its frequency. Unfortunately a migraine is not a once-in-a-lifetime thing. A person who suffers from migraine headaches will have them on a recurrent basis—although, of course, some people will have them more frequently than others.

3) Migraine seems to be inherited. In other words, you're not likely to be the only one in your family to suffer from migraine.

4) A migraine headache often involves only one side of the head. In fact, that's what the word "migraine" means—"half of the head."
5) A migraine may be accompanied by a number of other visual and neurological symptoms, including visual loss, seeing spots in front of the eyes, numbness of the face and hands, fainting, etc. These symptoms will be discussed in greater detail over the next few pages.

The pain and intensity of a migraine headache may be made worse by light and sound, so the victim may seek bedrest in a darkened room.

What causes a migraine headache?

Most headache specialists believe that a migraine headache results from a disturbance in the part of the brain that sends out messages to the brain's network of nerves and blood vessels. The disturbance primarily involves serotonin, a substance which apparently regulates many of the body's functions, including wakefulness and sleep. Serotonin is necessary for the human body to function, but it can cause trouble if the body's serotonin transmitter system does not function correctly. One headache specialist has likened this disturbance of the function of serotonin in the brain stem to a noisy computer chip. It has even been speculated that serotonin may be linked to certain kinds of mental illness—although this has nothing at all to do with migraine headaches. Serotonin, which originates from dietary tryptophan, is widely distributed in body tissues—most in the intestinal tract and about 8 per cent in blood platelets. Only 2 per cent is found in the brain. [61, 66]

What is "classical" migraine?

Classical migraine, also referred to as "migraine with aura" affects about 10 to 15 per cent of those who suffer from migraines. The person who suffers from this disorder usually is warned by a variety of visual symptoms—the "aura"—that a headache is about to occur. These visual symptoms, which usually last anywhere from 10 to 20 minutes, may include things like blinking lights, spots in front of the eyes, blind areas in the visual field, colored lights, partial blindness, tunnel vision, and lines that shimmer and dance in front of the eyes. Sometimes a crescent-shaped area surrounded by zig-zag lines may appear, shimmer and move across the visual field, getting bigger as it does so (see illustrations No. 1 and 2 on pages 11 and 13). Usually, the headache itself arrives a half-

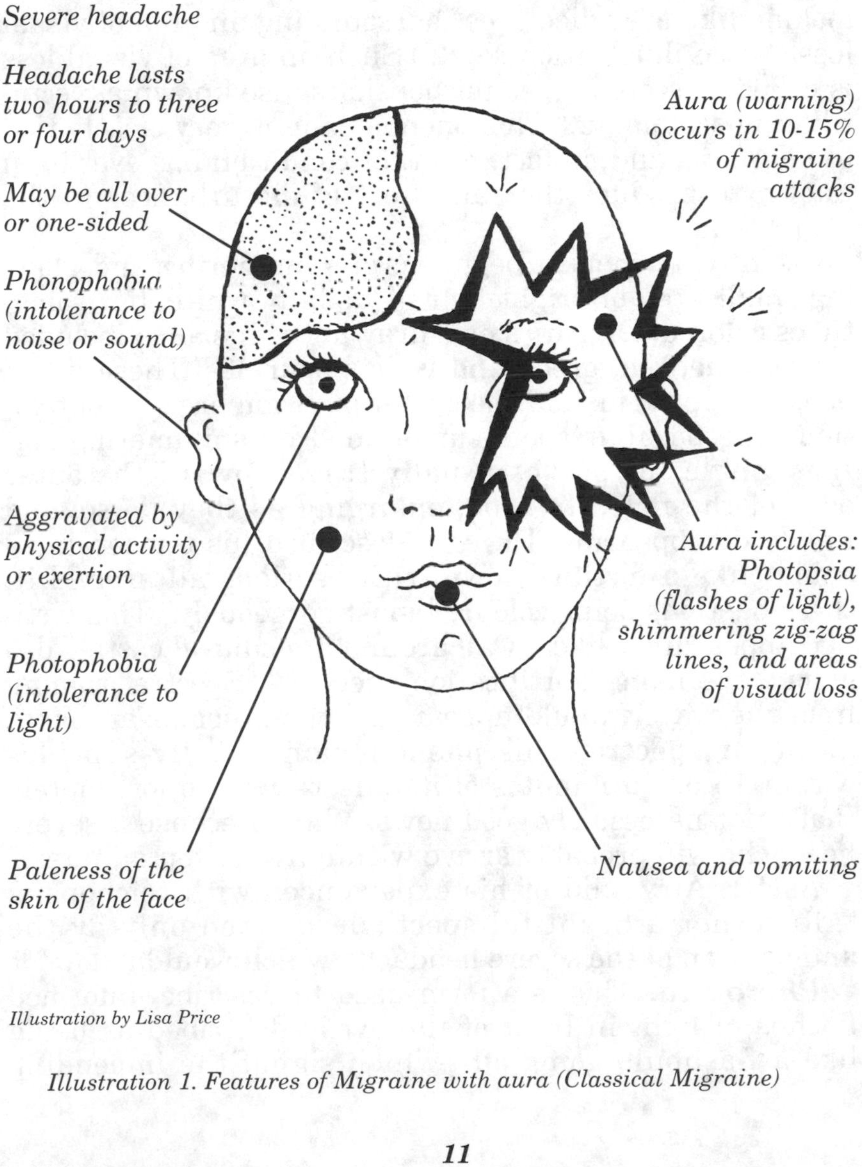

Severe headache

Headache lasts two hours to three or four days

Aura (warning) occurs in 10-15% of migraine attacks

May be all over or one-sided

Phonophobia (intolerance to noise or sound)

Aggravated by physical activity or exertion

Aura includes: Photopsia (flashes of light), shimmering zig-zag lines, and areas of visual loss

Photophobia (intolerance to light)

Paleness of the skin of the face

Nausea and vomiting

Illustration by Lisa Price

Illustration 1. Features of Migraine with aura (Classical Migraine)

hour or so after the visual symptoms go away—although in some instances they will continue during the headache. Some of the specific visual symptoms include:

Teichopsia (Walled Vision). Teichopsia is an often frightening visual disturbance which warns that a migraine attack is on its way. Teichopsia was thoroughly described in 1870 in a publication by Dr. Hubert Airy, who drew his visual aura in color. [39] Nearly a century prior to that, in 1778, Dr. Fothergill had also written about this phenomenon. Dr. Airy described teichopsia as looking like a "walled area" surrounding an area of visual loss. [39] (See illustration No. 2.) Such an area of visual loss is called a "scotoma," so teichopsia is also known as "scintillating scotomata." This phenomenon is very closely tied to migraine, and, in fact, no other condition has ever been known to produce the same sort of disturbances in the visual field.

Usually, teichopsia begins as a shimmering and glowing small area of bright lights—usually white, but sometimes colored. Dr. Airy's own drawing of his aura included white, blue, red, green and yellow sparkles. These lights usually appear just off the center of vision or point of fixation. The peculiar spots surrounded by shimmering zigzags, angles or prisms usually travel toward the outer edge of the field of vision, enlarging as they do so, and finally disappearing. Dr. Airy described his teichopsia as being "like a fortified town with bastions all around it, these bastions being coloured most gorgeously." This fortified appearance, like a wall around a medieval castle, also gained the name "fortification spectra." "Spectra" coming from the way it would appear and then disappear, like a ghost, or spectre. This phenomenon usually subsides within 15 or 20 minutes of its onset—but, unfortunately that's not necessarily good news. Why? Because a severe headache will probably arrive within five or ten minutes.

As Dr. Airy said of his experiences with teichopsia: "Altogether a beautiful spectacle marred only by the anticipation of the severe headache which would follow." [39]

Photopsia. This is a term used to describe unformed flashes of light in front of the eyes—described as being like a flashbulb going off—which signal the impending

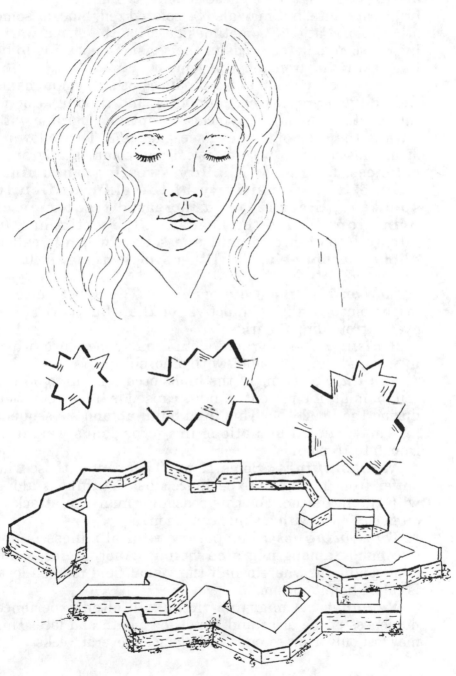

Illustration by Lisa Price

Illustration 2. Typical aura of Fortification Spectra of Migraine

arrival of a migraine. These flashes of light are usually bright or white, but may also be colored red, blue, or some other color. Patients sometimes describe the visual warnings of scotomata as areas in their vision appearing to be like heat rising from a hot pavement.

A classical migraine also produces other symptoms as well; difficulty speaking, numbness and tingling around the mouth or hands. A typical example of migraine with aura is the case of 'James' (see page 17). The following symptoms occur in both classical and common migraine: **coldness**, **fatigue**, **irritability, sweating**, **abdominal pain**, extreme **sensitivity of the skin**, **difficulty speaking**, **diarrhea**, and increased **frequency of urination**. During the headache, the victim has an intense intolerance to light and sound, which is called **phonophotophobia**. [18, 59, 61] Other symptoms may include:

Subconjunctival hemorrhage: The appearance of bright blood in the conjunctiva, or the white part of the eyes surrounding the iris.

Bruising: The migraine victim may experience bruising around the eyes, along with a nosebleed.

Swelling: Swelling of the limbs occurs in up to 95 per cent of migraine patients, and is caused by fluid retention during the headache. This fluid build up and subsequent loss may cause fluctuations in the patient's weight of from 5 to 15 pounds.

Nasal stuffiness: Some 10 to 20 per cent of those who suffer from migraine experience nasal stuffiness along with the headache. For this reason, a migraine attack is often confused with a sinus condition.

Total blindness: Temporary total blindness is not uncommon among migraine victims. Another, less common condition, wherein half the visual field may be lost, is called hemianopsia.

Numbness: A migraine victim will often experience numbness of the arms and hands, or mouth and face. This may last only a few seconds, or as long as several weeks. [18, 61]

What is "common" migraine?

Common migraine headache is that which occurs without any of the visual or other neurological symptoms that accompany classical migraine, although there may be various warning signals up to 24 hours before the onset of the headache. This period of warning—which doctors call the "prodrome,"—may include irritability, craving for certain foods (especially chocolate and other sweets), and excessive yawning, mentioned in Dr. Liveing's book in 1873, or difficulty with speech.[39] Other than the lack of the aura, the two headaches are basically the same: very painful, accompanied by nausea and vomiting, and aggravated by exposure to light and sound or by exertion.[18, 61] Typical cases of migraine without aura, or common migraine, are those of 'Tammy,' 'Audra,' and 'Beth' (see pages 18, 19 and 20 and illustration No. 3).

How long will a migraine last?

Unfortunately, a migraine headache usually lasts for several hours—occasionally even up to 72 hours or longer. After the headache passes, the victim will feel tired and washed out and is also likely to experience soreness and tenderness of the scalp.[18, 61]

What if I faint? Is that a sign something else is wrong?

Fainting is a fairly common symptom among migraine sufferers. In fact, about 10 per cent of migraine victims will faint with the onset of the headache. This does not generally indicate that anything else is wrong.[61]

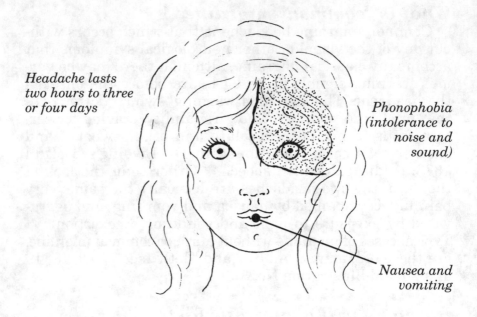

Headache lasts two hours to three or four days

Phonophobia (intolerance to noise and sound)

Nausea and vomiting

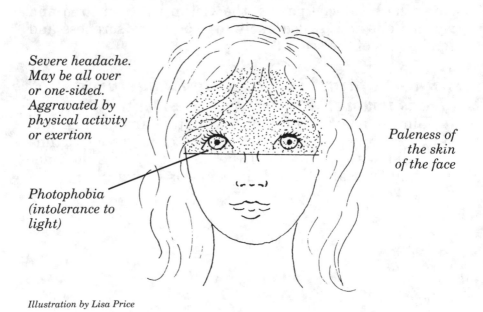

Severe headache. May be all over or one-sided. Aggravated by physical activity or exertion

Paleness of the skin of the face

Photophobia (intolerance to light)

Illustration by Lisa Price

Illustration 3. Migraine without aura (Common Migraine)

"James"

Headache History

James, age fifty-two, had experienced severe headache at least once a month lasting about three days each time. The headaches were almost always preceded by "flashing lights" and "crinkle-like star figures" in his vision, lasting fifteen to twenty minutes. Other symptoms included temporary visual loss and numbness in his left hand and arm. Following this he had a dull headache for another day, increased pain when bending over, and sensitivity to bright light and noise.

Previous Treatment

Before visiting me, James' treatment included simple Tylenol® and aspirin with minimal relief.

Neurological exam, blood pressure and lab results were all normal.

My Diagnosis

James was diagnosed as having Migraine With Typical Aura (Classical Migraine).

Effective Treatment

Verapamil, a calcium channel blocker, was prescribed to prevent headaches, and James was instructed to take two Cafergot® tablets at onset of visual symptoms plus Reglan® to control nausea.

Progress

After a month of continued headache, James' dosage of verapamil was increased. This provided him with headache prevention for the first time in ten years. Follow-up several months later revealed that James remained headache free.

"Tammy"

Headache History
Thirty-four-year-old Tammy came to us with left-sided headache for the past two years. She never smiled or laughed, preferred being by herself, and hardly ate one meal a day. Once or twice a month she had more severe throbbing headaches for up to thirty-six hours which she called "migraine." Tammy experienced nausea and vomiting, intolerance to light and sound, dizziness, tearing, and numbness of the arms. At times she had sharp stabs of left-sided head pain. More severe headaches seemed to be brought about by stress, exertion, oversleeping, coughing, chewing, stooping, and even talking. She felt tired, nervous, and cold, and could not sleep. She suffered from pain in her back and joints. Her mother and sister also had headaches. She smoked a pack of cigarettes a day. Tammy had to take Xanax® and Tylenol® just to get some sleep. On examination, she was tender on the left side of the neck. A trigger point was injected with local anesthetic and steroid for relief. CT brain scan and laboratory tests were normal.

My Diagnosis
Migraine Without Aura.

Effective Treatment
She was placed on a preventive program of diet, verapamil, and amitriptyline. She was allowed to take Fiorinal® for more severe headaches, never more than two days a week. For her severest headache, she was instructed to use dihydroergotamine (or DHE45®) and Reglan® by self-injection.

Progress
She was so improved after a month that she could hardly believe it. Her constant headache was gone. Amazingly, Tammy had only three minor headaches relieved by Fiorinal® not requiring any injection of dihydroergotamine. She now enjoys people, "felt wonderful", and exclaimed, "It's wonderful to be pain free!"

"Audra"

Headache History

Audra was sixty-three when she came to us in early February, 1993. For two years she had had dull, burning, constant left-sided head pain which seemed to involve the left ear, left temple, and left forehead. The pain increased with chewing and with rainy, damp weather. She sometimes had the sensation of feeling numb and dizzy. She had been prescribed a brace for suspected TMJ dysfunction. She was tired, could not sleep, was depressed, had joint pains, numbness of her hands, problems in her sex life, and felt cold. She saw a neurologist at a university clinic, and a CT and MRI brain scan were both normal. She also had colitis and was taking sulfasalazine.

Her neurological examination, blood pressure, EEG and lab tests were normal.

My Diagnosis

Migraine Without Aura.

Effective Treatment

Indocin® was tried by suppository, since she could not take Indocin by mouth because of her intestinal problems. Indocin® provided no relief. She was placed on amitriptyline, Inderal®, and Anaprox® along with a headache diet. Anaprox® produced tingling of her limbs and was stopped. She did not improve after a month and was hospitalized for treatment with intravenous dihydroergotamine and Compazine®. Within a few days, she became completely headache free and was discharged on dihydroergotamine by sustained release capsules.

Progress

She remains headache free.

"Beth"

Headache History

Beth, age thirty-two, had a history of severe headaches lasting from six hours to two and a half weeks...each episode of pain occurred every month or two. Her pain occurred mostly in the forehead radiating to the back and right side of the head. Sometimes her entire head would hurt. Headaches would always occur one or two days immediately prior to her menstrual periods. Headaches were throbbing, tight and pressure-like, with nausea and vomiting. With headaches came sleeplessness, intolerance to light and sounds, neck stiffness, and general numbness.

Neurological exam, blood pressure, lab tests, CT scan and EEG were all normal.

Previous Treatment

A number of medications were tried by her physician... including Midrin®, Lortab®, Stadol®, Demerol®, and Cafergot® which only seemed to dull the pain. Inderal® was taken for a short time without benefit.

My Diagnosis

Migraine Without Aura.

Effective Treatment

Beth was advised to stop taking over-the-counter medications and to reduce her alcohol and cigarette usage. Inderal® and nortriptyline were given to prevent headaches. Self injections of DHE45® were prescribed for breakthrough headaches along with Reglan® tablets to prevent nausea.

Progress

After one month, Beth's headaches continued but were less severe. The Inderal® and nortriptyline dosages were increased, and Beth became headache free over a four month period. According to Beth, "My doctor has given me my life back." She continues to do well on Inderal® and nortriptyline.

What is a "migraine equivalent?"

A migraine equivalent is what happens when a person has all of the visual warning symptoms of a classical migraine—the spots in front of the eyes, the colored lights, partial blindness, etc.—but without the headache itself. The migraine equivalent seems to occur more frequently in men who are over the age of 60, and may be quite frightening, since the victim may feel that a stroke is about to occur. Actually, a migraine equivalent is not serious, and usually lasts for no more than 20 or 30 minutes. At the same time, the person who suffers from a migraine equivalent should report the episode to his doctor, just to rule out any other cause of the episode. [18, 61]

Is there really a "migraine personality?"

No...not really. At one time it was thought that migraine headaches were associated with a tendency to be a perfectionist. A person who was inflexible, demanding, compulsive, and especially demanding of himself, was felt to be prone to migraine headaches.

However, in the last few years, the thinking of most headache specialists on this subject has changed. Numerous psychological studies of migraine sufferers have been done, and no clear personality patterns have emerged. It now appears that a tendency to suffer from migraine is inherited, and not associated with any specific personality type. Migraine headache patients are no more perfectionistic or compulsive than those who do not suffer from migraine. [18, 61]

It may be small consolation during the pain of a migraine headache, but at least the migraine sufferer can now know that he isn't "responsible" for his headache. His personality doesn't really have a great deal to do with it.

But can't stress bring on a migraine?

Yes, it is true that emotional stress is often involved with the onset of a migraine headache. In fact, about half of all migraine victims report that they suffered their first such headaches during a time of stress or worry.

However, further studies have shown that a migraine headache results principally from biological and not emotional factors. In other words, the person who has inherited a tendency to suffer from migraines may be more prone to get them during times of stress or worry. But this does not mean that worry or stress can necessarily produce a migraine headache in anyone. Nor is it true that stress is always the primary trigger of a migraine headache. Studies have also shown that there is a pronounced tendency for these headaches to develop in the "letdown" of relaxation immediately after stressful periods. [18, 59, 61]

So again, stress and worry may be considered "trigger factors" in generating migraine headaches, but they are not the basic cause.

What do you mean by "trigger factors?"

Headaches can be brought on by several different factors, all of which are referred to as "trigger factors."

One such trigger factor is stress. Another trigger factor may be menstruation.

Some foods may trigger headaches, especially alcohol, chocolate, aged cheeses, caffeine, certain kinds of nuts, nitrites, and nitrates.

A change in the weather or the changing of seasons may also trigger a headache. So can changes in schedule and sleeping patterns, changes in diet, a sudden change of altitude, and so on.

Other trigger factors include: bright or flickering lights, strong odors, times of intense activity, any loss such as death, separation or divorce, or any crisis in a person's personal life.

When you think of the head—and brain—as the body's control center, it's easy to see why the common result of these activities is a headache—and more specifically, a migraine in those who are prone to having them. Any occurrence that can leave you feeling "out of sync" or "off-balance," can put stress on the headache sufferer, and result in a headache. [59, 61, 72]

But again, it's worth mentioning that it is not necessarily true that any of these things can produce a headache, unless the person has inherited a tendency to have headaches.

What is "menstrual migraine?"

As was mentioned earlier, three-fourths of those who suffer from migraine headaches are women, and many of these get such headaches only right before, during, or a day or two after their periods. In these women, the migraine seems to be directly related to a lessening of the amount of the female hormone estrogen in the body during the time of menstruation. Women who suffer from these menstrual headaches seem to be extremely vulnerable to certain headache triggers, such as the letdown after stress, stress itself, certain foods, alcohol, fatigue, loss of sleep, or oversleeping. [20, 61, 72]

One thing that seems to help prevent such headaches is to increase the amount of estrogen in the body, and a simple way to do this is to wear an estrogen patch for a few days before and during the menstrual period. [72] We'll talk more about treatment for this and other types of headaches in Part Four of this book.

What is "childhood migraine?"

Childhood migraine is just what it sounds like—a migraine headache suffered by a child.

Childhood migraine is the most common cause of headache in children—but the good news is that someone who suffers from migraine as a child will not necessarily continue to suffer from such attacks throughout his life. It's not at all uncommon for a cycle of frequent and severe headaches to last for about six months and then disappear; however, if the child's headaches are accompanied by bouts of nausea or vomiting, there is a 75 per cent chance that he will suffer from typical migraine headaches later in life.

While childhood migraines are similar to those suffered by adults, there are some notable differences. For example, about 60 per cent of those who suffer from childhood migraine are boys, whereas, as was mentioned earlier, 75 per cent of adult migraine victims are women. Another difference is that childhood migraines generally don't last as long as the "adult version." They may last no more than 15 minutes and rarely persist for more than 12 hours. Another significant feature of childhood migraine is that it may be accompanied by severe abdominal pain. In fact, there is increasing evidence that children who suffer from periodic severe stomach pain also may actually be experiencing migraine attacks! Childhood migraine also may be accompanied by dizziness, or sleep disturbances such as bed-wetting, nightmares, and episodes of sleepwalking.

Several trigger factors may come into play in the onset of a childhood migraine. These include: coming out of a darkened place (such as a movie theater) into bright sunlight, physical exertion, hunger, noise, cold weather, or stress at school. [18, 59, 61] (See the case of 'Jason' on page 25 as a typical example of childhood migraine.)

"Jason"

Headache History

Jason, age six, came to us in early June, 1993, with headaches about once a week for two years. His parents described Jason's headaches as "just a headache," relieved by Tylenol®. However, about twice a month, or even more frequently, he had more severe headache lasting up to three hours, with nausea and vomiting, so that he would sleep for relief. Jason described his headache as throbbing and in the right forehead, interfering with his play. His mother said that he was sensitive to light and sound. Fatigue and missing a meal might precipitate headache. Jason's mother, maternal grandmother, and grandfather all had headaches. His examination and EEG were normal.

Previous Treatment

Tylenol® with codeine had been given by another physician.

My Diagnosis

Childhood Migraine.

Effective Treatment

Jason was placed on a low tyramine, low caffeine diet and cyproheptadine at bedtime as a preventive. For headache, he was to use Tylenol® by tablet or suppository. After four weeks on cyproheptadine, he had had no severe headaches with vomiting. He had several minor headaches which responded to Tylenol®.

What is "Alice in Wonderland" syndrome?

This is a name for an uncommon type of visual distortion produced by the "aura" of a classical migraine. The technical name for this distortion is "metamorphopsia." Lewis Carroll, the author of *Alice's Adventures in Wonderland*, suffered from such headaches, and it is widely believed that the "metamorphopsia" he experienced apparently gave Carroll the idea for many of the bizarre characters in his classic story (see illustration No. 4 on page 27). If that is so, it may be the only time in history that anyone ever profited from having a migraine headache! It's also easy to see why "Alice in Wonderland Syndrome" would be the commonly used term, instead of a hard-to-pronounce and even harder-to-spell word like "metamorphopsia." [19]

As you can imagine, metamorphopsia, with its distortions and hallucinations, can be quite frightening—probably similar to taking a "bad trip" on a hallucinogenic drug, but it can be even more frightening because the victim hasn't done anything to bring it on. The good news is that it usually doesn't last long—maybe 20 minutes or so—but the bad news—worse than the Alice in Wonderland syndrome itself—is that a migraine is on its way.

What is basilar migraine?

Basilar migraine frequently attacks teenage girls and women under the age of 35, and may be precipitated by minor head trauma. This disorder includes a number of striking symptoms, including nausea or vomiting, whirling dizziness or vertigo, slurred speech, difficulty walking, double vision, and temporary blindness. Altered consciousness may occur within 30 minutes after the onset of an attack, and the patient will have a severe, throbbing headache, usually in the back of the head. The victim will usually go to sleep within 30 minutes after the onset of symptoms, and sleep will terminate the attack. Upon awakening, the patient may experience tenderness of the scalp. The case of Michelle (on page 29) is a typical example of basilar migraine and its response to Tegretol®. [18, 61]

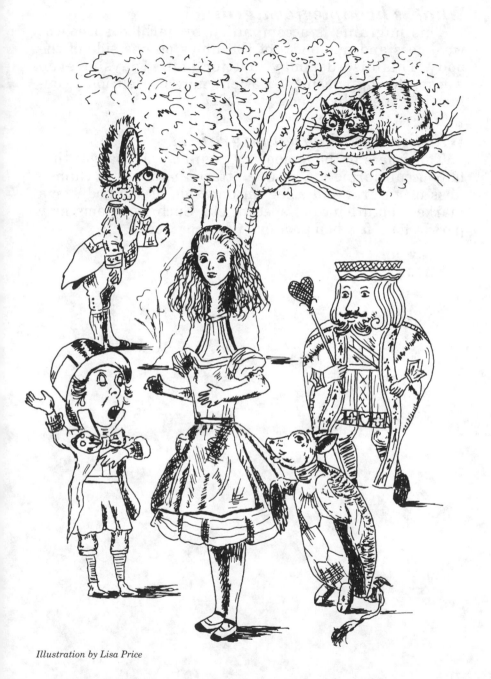

Illustration by Lisa Price

Illustration 4. Lewis Carroll likely had Metamorphopsia with distorted figures in his vision giving him the idea for the characters in <u>Alice's Adventures in Wonderland</u>.

What is hemiplegic migraine?

This migraine is accompanied by garbled speech or weakness and numbness of the limbs on one side of the body. This disorder may last for hours, days or even weeks, during which the patient may be delirious, confused or "mentally cloudy." [18,61]

What is complicated migraine?

This refers to the temporary neurological changes that may occur during a migraine attack: paralysis or clumsiness of an arm and a leg on one side of the body, or a marked disturbance of speech, etc. Such symptoms may persist for a few hours, or even days or weeks. [18, 61]

"Michelle"

Headache History

This twenty-four-year-old lady had been having incapacitating headaches since she was 19—usually about once a month and frequently on Sunday afternoons. They would begin with unusual neurological symptoms such as "feeling that she was not in herself." Michelle would then experience half-vision or yellow vision, which she described as being like paint or spots in front of her eyes, and then complete blindness, which she called "black vision." She also experienced buzzing in the ears and a marked intensification of sounds. She would become numb throughout her body, especially in the cheeks and lips, and often had the sensation that her "throat would go to sleep," which, in turn, caused her to feel that she could not breathe and was going to suffocate. The difficulty with her throat also rendered her unable to speak. The headache itself was described as burning and throbbing and was located in the crown and back part of the head. It brought with it increased sensitivity to light, and was accompanied by nausea and vomiting. Within about 30 minutes she would go to sleep for several hours, during which time the attack would terminate. When she awoke, soreness of her head was the only aftereffect. Michelle reported that her mother also suffered from severe headaches.

Previous Treatment

Dilantin® was tried, but was discontinued because it produced a generalized skin rash and fever, even though she had no attacks during the three weeks she was on that medication. During this time she was also tired, nervous, and had frequent fainting spells. Inderal®, verapamil, and Bellergal® had not helped.

Laboratory tests, including a CT brain scan and EEG, were normal. Her prolactin level was normal, and her blood pressure was 120/75. Noteworthy is the fact that she had begun lactating three or four months previously, even though her only child was now four years old, and she had not breast-fed for several years. During this time she continued to have regular menstrual periods.

My Diagnosis
Basilar Migraine along with persistent lactation.

Effective Treatment
Bromocriptine was begun, but produced nausea and dizziness and had to be stopped. However, the lactation stopped and did not recur. Tegretol ® was then begun twice daily. Eighteen days later Michelle was clearly better. She was seen again a month later, and reported that she had experienced no further severe attacks and had only occasional minor headaches which responded to Midrin®.

THE MOTHER OF ALL HEADACHES: THE MIGRAINE

A LOOK AT OTHER TYPES AND CAUSES OF HEADACHES

· ·

There are actually dozens of different types of headaches that may be brought on by dozens of different causes. While it would be impossible to discuss every single type of headache in a book like this one, it is possible to talk about some of the less common types of headaches and causes.

Again, what follows are some of the headache-related questions that are asked by patients at the Ford Headache Clinic.

Can a headache be the sign of a brain tumor?

Yes, a chronic headache can, in fact, be caused by a brain tumor...but the vast majority of headaches have far less ominous sources. If you are afraid that you might be suffering from a brain tumor, then by all means get to a doctor for a checkup. But don't think that a prolonged or recurring headache is by any means a sure sign that you are suffering from a brain tumor.

Usually, headache pain produced by a brain tumor or abscess is of recent origin and tends to increase in severity and frequency. Pain may be worse when the victim is lying down and may be very severe upon first awakening in the morning. Typically, a headache brought on by a brain tumor is dull, doesn't throb, and may be made worse by exertion or change of position.

This type of headache is frequently accompanied by nausea and vomiting—which may precede the headache by several days or weeks. Two-thirds of children who suffer from brain tumors are either awakened during the night by headaches or complain of severe headaches upon first arising in the morning.

Again…it should be repeated that not one of these symptoms—or even all of these symptoms combined—is a sure sign that someone is suffering from a brain tumor. But if you have any concerns, you should express them to your doctor. [59]

What is "cluster headache?"

Cluster headache is actually more painful than a migraine, but also, thankfully, much shorter. Cluster headache may build in intensity for 5 to 10 minutes or so and then persist for anywhere from 20 minutes to two hours. The reason they are called "cluster" headaches is that they seem to attack in bunches. In other words, the victim may experience a number of these short, severe headaches over a period of weeks or months. This will be followed by a relatively long headache free period—and then another "cluster" of attacks. In some instances patients may have daily cluster headaches without a remission, or break, in the cycle. This form is called chronic cluster headache.

Interestingly enough, cluster headaches almost always occur in men—at a ratio of about seven to one—whereas women are three times more likely than men to suffer from migraine. It is not really understood why cluster headaches are so much more likely to strike males than females—but it is an undisputed fact.

Cluster headaches—which occur in less than one per cent of the population—always occur on the same side of the victim's head, generally at the same time of the day or night, and in one specific area, such as the eye socket or the temple. Patients have described the pain as feeling "like a hot poker behind the eye." This severe pain is often accompanied by tearing, a runny nose, stuffiness of the nostril on the side of the headache, redness of the affected eye, drooping of the eyelid, or the bulging out of veins in the scalp or temple.

The person who suffers from cluster headaches will typically pace back and forth, as if he's trying to outrun the pain. It hurts too much to just "lie there." This is the exact opposite behavior of the migraine victim, who is likely to lie quietly curled up in bed in a darkened, quiet room. [18, 34, 61] (See illustration No. 5, and see the case histories of 'Farris' and 'Roland' on Pages 97 and 98.)

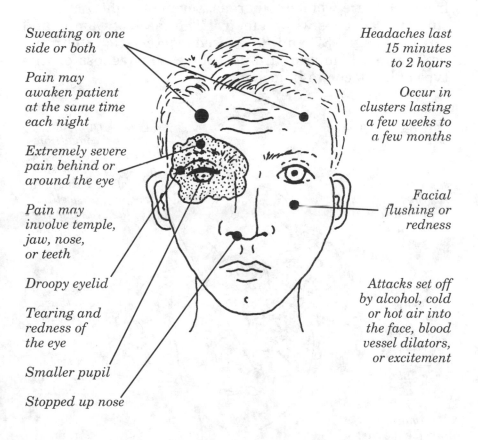

Sweating on one side or both

Pain may awaken patient at the same time each night

Extremely severe pain behind or around the eye

Pain may involve temple, jaw, nose, or teeth

Droopy eyelid

Tearing and redness of the eye

Smaller pupil

Stopped up nose

Headaches last 15 minutes to 2 hours

Occur in clusters lasting a few weeks to a few months

Facial flushing or redness

Attacks set off by alcohol, cold or hot air into the face, blood vessel dilators, or excitement

Illustration by Lisa Price

Illustration 5. Cluster Headache

What is "chronic paroxysmal hemicrania?"

Chronic paroxysmal hemicrania is a rare variation of cluster headache. It involves 10 to 20 brief but intense localized head pains in the space of a single day. These attacks are sometimes brought on by movement of the head or neck. The pain is usually felt on only one side of the head and focused around the eye, ear, or back of the head (see illustration No. 6). These headaches are somewhat similar to cluster headaches already discussed. The major differences are that headaches associated with chronic paroxysmal hemicrania are usually much shorter than cluster headaches and that most of those who suffer from them are women, whereas, seven of eight victims of cluster headaches will be men. [74] The cases of Camile and Sara on pages 37 and 38 are characteristic of chronic paroxysmal hemicrania, and the responsiveness of this type of headache to Indocin®.

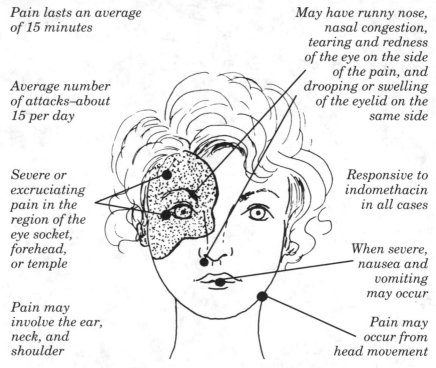

Pain lasts an average of 15 minutes

May have runny nose, nasal congestion, tearing and redness of the eye on the side of the pain, and drooping or swelling of the eyelid on the same side

Average number of attacks–about 15 per day

Severe or excruciating pain in the region of the eye socket, forehead, or temple

Responsive to indomethacin in all cases

When severe, nausea and vomiting may occur

Pain may involve the ear, neck, and shoulder

Pain may occur from head movement

Illustration by Lisa Price

Illustration 6. Chronic Paroxysmal Hemicrania (One-sided jabbing head pains in women)

"Camile"

Headache History

Camile, age thirty-five, injured her neck in an automobile accident eight months previously. She subsequently began to experience recurring left-sided headaches. Stabbing, severe pains lasting ten to thirty minutes occurred three to five times a day, even during sleep. Her headaches were worsened by menstruation, certain foods, stress, stooping, odors, and alcohol.

Neurological exam, lab studies, MRI scan and EEG were all normal.

My Diagnosis

Chronic Paroxysmal Hemicrania.

Effective Treatment

A daily dosage of Indocin® was prescribed. She continued to experience occasional breakthrough headaches after six months, and her dosage of Indocin® was increased.

Camile's headaches dramatically stopped when she began taking Indocin®. When last examined, Camile's headaches were under control except when she experienced high stress levels.

"Sara"

Headache History

Sara came to us at age fifty-nine in the summer of 1990 with a history of headaches beginning in her early forties. She had been seen by another neurologist in 1972 and had been diagnosed as having cluster headaches. These groups of headaches occurred about every six months with repeated headache attacks which would last a month or six weeks at a time. Her headaches occurred as often as every two hours with severe pain in the right temple and right eye socket with tearing and redness of the right eye along with nasal stuffiness and runny nose on the right. Headaches lasted thirty to forty-five minutes occurring night and day up to six times within twenty-four hours.

Previous Treatment

She had taken a number of medications in large amounts including Bufferin® up to twelve tablets per day, injections of Demerol®, Tylenol®, Darvon®, codeine, Sansert®, Periactin®, ibuprofen, and lithium carbonate, all without benefit. She had also been given a short course of prednisone and lithium carbonate along with ergotamine tartrate by inhalation, none of which helped her.

Her examination and laboratory tests, CT brain scan, EEG, and thermogram were normal. Blood pressure was 120/80.

My Diagnosis

Chronic Paroxysmal Hemicrania.

Effective Treatment

The patient was taken off all analgesics and was begun on Indocin® three times per day. In a few days the patient had no headaches at all, and Indocin® was decreased to only once or twice a day.

The patient was seen again in six months and was still headache free. On her last visit in the summer of 1993, she had remained headache free simply by taking Indocin®, usually once a day.

What is "hemicrania continua?"

This rare and unusual headache disorder may last for several years and is characterized by a continuous, dull ache on one side of the head—along with jabbing, ice-pick-like pains which may be brought about by physical exertion. In other words, "hemicrania continua" might be considered a "two-fisted" sort of adversary that combines into one painful experience some of the worst attributes of other types of headaches! (See illustration No. 7.)

The intense pains of hemicrania continua may last anywhere from 5 to 45 minutes and may occur several times throughout the day—and night. Sometimes these pains may be accompanied by nausea and sensitivity to light. This type of headache afflicts people of various ages, from adolescence on, and seems to have no preference between males and females. The arthritis drug indomethacin is always an effective remedy for those who suffer from these headaches. [18, 59, 72, 75] The case of Roanna on page 40 illustrates hemicrania continua's responsiveness to indomethacin.

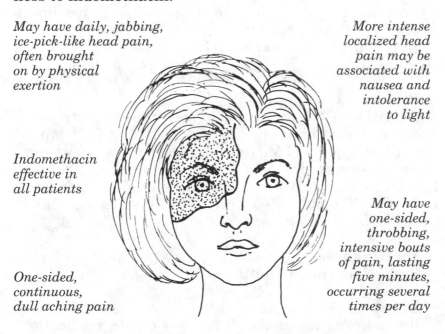

May have daily, jabbing, ice-pick-like head pain, often brought on by physical exertion

More intense localized head pain may be associated with nausea and intolerance to light

Indomethacin effective in all patients

May have one-sided, throbbing, intensive bouts of pain, lasting five minutes, occurring several times per day

One-sided, continuous, dull aching pain

Illustration by Lisa Price

Illustration 7. Hemicrania Continua (Constant one-sided head pain)

"Roanna"

Headache History

A thirty-two-year-old mother of two, Roanna came to our practice after six years of constant, dull, daily headache. Ninety percent of her pain occurred on the right side of her head...sharp, jabbing, "ice-pick-like" pain just above the right ear. Occasional severe, throbbing head pain along with sensitivity to light and sound would last up to a week...interfering with daily activities and causing irritability, difficulty in sleeping, early morning awakening, and neck stiffness.

Fatigue, stress, coughing, chewing, and talking seemed to make the pain worse.

Other symptoms included persistent diarrhea following gall bladder surgery (she was unable to lose weight, however). She was also troubled by depression, tiredness, nervousness, problems in her sex life, and heartburn. She perspired excessively and had poor appetite, heart palpitations, and generally felt ill.

Roanna neither smoked nor drank alcohol...her brother also experienced headache.

Her neurological examination, blood pressure, lab studies, EEG, and CT scan of the brain were all normal.

Previous Treatment

A previous CT brain scan had been reported as normal. Roanna's physician treated her with a splint for temporomandibular joint (TMJ) problems along with Valium® three times each day plus Tylox®, Voltaren® and Xanax®. Early medication treatment also included Percodan®, Darvocet®, Fiorinal®, Mepergan®, Midrin®, Reglan®, Advil®, Orudis®, Naprosyn®, Anaprox®, Ergostat®, and Cafergot®.

My Diagnosis

Right Hemicrania Continua.

Effective Treatment

Roanna was taken off all analgesic pain medications slowly over the next month. Xanax® was discontinued, and the Valium® dosage was reduced. She was also given Indocin® three times daily for pain.

Progress
A month later, Roanna became headache free by taking Indocin® twice each day plus Zantac® for heartburn.

What is an "orgasmic" headache?

Now we're back to the old line, "Not tonight dear, I have a headache." The actual fact is that sexual intercourse gives some people a headache! This is similar to a headache brought on by exertion or an intense coughing spell.

Although in some patients headache occurs frequently with sexual activity, in most the occurrence of headache is infrequent and completely unpredictable. Most of the time headache is relatively severe and located in the front or back of the head. It may be explosive or throbbing or like a "thunderclap." This usually begins shortly before or just at the time of reaching a climax. The headache may last a few minutes or may sometimes linger as a dull headache for a couple of days. Sometimes it is difficult or impossible to be certain this type thunderclap headache associated with lovemaking is not related to rupture of an aneurysm or even an unruptured aneurysm as the cause. Surely, if vomiting or severe headache lasts more than twenty-four hours, investigation for aneurysm with an MR angiogram or four-vessel arteriogram may be necessary to be certain an aneurysm is not the cause. Some patients with this problem give a history of hypertension, a strong family history of migraine, or even a prior history of migraine. You should see your doctor, who may refer you to a neurologist or neurosurgeon, or a headache specialist, to rule out the possibility of an underlying organic cause, such as ruptured or unruptured aneurysm.

Once that has been done, there is good news. A tendency to this type of headache is no reason for a husband and wife to avoid intimacy. There are treatments available. This type of headache is particularly sensitive to indomethacin, the nonsteroidal anti-inflammatory drug or arthritic medicine. [18, 41, 61, 71]

What is "thunderclap" headache?

"Thunderclap" headache may be a warning that something is seriously wrong. It derives its name from the fact that it comes on with extreme suddenness and intensity—like a clap of thunder—and it often occurs a few days or weeks prior to the occurrence of a cerebral hemorrhage. In fact, about half the victims of such a hemor-rhage will experience a thunderclap headache a few days or weeks before the hemorrhage itself. If more victims of thunderclap headache would seek immediate medical attention, certainly fewer of them would die or suffer from paralysis or other permanent disabilities.

This type of headache is brought on by the leaking of blood into the spinal fluid as a blood vessel begins to rup-ture. If the situation is diagnosed and treated in time, severe damage can often be prevented.

You might think of it as like noticing that one of the tires on your car is bad. If you change the tire, you have nothing to worry about. But if you continue to drive on it, you're likely to have a blowout and even a severe and potentially fatal accident.

If you are not prone to headaches, and suddenly find yourself hit by intense pain, you should see your doctor, headache specialist, or neurological consultant as quickly as possible. He can use an arteriogram, or angiogram, an X-ray procedure which outlines arteries and veins inside the head, to tell if there is a serious problem. [16, 18, 61]

What is "ice-pick" head pain?

This is a jabbing or jolting pain which has been described as being stuck with an "ice-pick"—thus, its name. Those who suffer from this kind of headache have also described them as "needle-like," or "a sharp pin-prick," or like "being stuck with a nail."

Ice-pick head pains are experienced by about 40 per cent of those who suffer from migraine attacks, and more than half of these report that they experience the pains at least once a month. Ice-pick pains usually occur in the temples and the areas around the eyes.

The majority of those who suffer from ice-pick headaches report that they have single, isolated jabs or jolts of pain, although some say they experience repeated volleys or jabs of these stabbing pains. Victims of this type of headache can often get relief from the non-steroidal arthritic medication, indomethacin. [18, 61, 62, 67]

At this point, the question may arise, "But what if I can't tell the difference between a thunderclap headache and an ice-pick headache, or between a migraine and a cluster headache?" The answer to that question is the old cliche, "It's always better to be safe than sorry." If you're not sure what's going on in your head, the best thing to do is pay a visit to your doctor or a headache specialist just to make sure there is nothing seriously wrong.

What is "hot dog" headache?

Once again, this headache is just what it sounds like— one that is brought on by the eating of a hot dog or other cured-meat product. It is believed that this type of headache is brought on by the nitrites and nitrates that are used to cure and preserve such meats. The pain in this type of headache may be in the temple or forehead and may seem to pulsate. A headache that is the result of eating a hot dog may be accompanied by redness of the face.

U.S. government regulations limit the amount of nitrite levels to 200 milligrams per kilogram of meat, but even that is enough to cause an intense headache in someone who is sensitive to nitrites. [27, 61]

What is "Chinese restaurant syndrome?"

Chinese restaurant syndrome is headache—and other symptoms—brought on by the ingestion of monosodium glutamate (MSG). The symptoms usually arise about 20 minutes after the food with MSG is eaten, and nearly one-third of those who eat in Chinese restaurants suffer from this syndrome. If you are especially fond of Chinese food, but can't seem to eat it without getting a headache, one answer is to ask your waitress if your food can be prepared without the use of MSG. Many restaurants will be able to comply with this request.

Generally, Chinese restaurant syndrome is made worse by the ingestion of alcohol.

It's not really known why MSG produces a severe reaction in some people, but the symptoms it produces may include in addition to head pain, tightness of the face, dizziness, diarrhea, nausea, and abdominal cramping. Bear in mind that MSG is not used exclusively in Chinese food. It may also be found in other foods—particularly in frozen foods. [61]

What other food might be the source of a headache?

There are a number of foods and beverages that can produce headaches in those that are especially sensitive to specific foods.

For example, alcoholic beverages such as wine and beer contain chemicals such as tyramine and phenylethylamine which can produce headaches (and, of course, so can the alcohol itself). Citrus fruits, chocolates, and dairy products may contain octopamine, phenylethylamine, and tyramine, which can trigger a migraine attack.

As we've already seen, nitrites, which are used in the curing process of meats such as bacon and ham, may also precipitate migraine attacks. Other common culprits? monosodium glutamate; the synthetic sweetener aspartame; anything pickled, fermented or marinated; nuts, including peanut butter; and broad beans.

But remember, this is by no means meant to be a complete list of foods that can bring on headaches. A complete list of foods appears later. [19, 38, 46, 53, 76]

Why do I get a headache when I eat ice cream?

Ice cream headache is an intense, but very brief pain, usually centered in the forehead, and it is brought on by eating ice cream or quickly gulping iced drinks—such as Slurpees or frozen margaritas. What is happening, really, is that your body is saying, "Hey...that's too cold! Slow down!" This headache is more likely to occur if you are overheated or have been exercising in hot weather. For example, if you're working in your yard on a hot day and then step inside your house for a refreshing glass of ice-cold water, you may be setting yourself up for an ice cream headache.

Generally, the pain in this type of headache reaches its peak 30 to 60 seconds after exposure to cold food or drink and then will quickly subside. Studies have shown that ice cream headache occurs in 90 per cent of patients who suffer from migraine, but in only about 30 per cent of the rest of the population. [61, 62]

What is "tension headache?"

For years, it was believed that headaches could be brought on by contraction of the muscles in the head or neck caused by stress or tension. But several studies have failed to confirm this muscle contraction.

It is now generally believed by many headache specialists that what used to be referred to as muscle contraction "tension headache" is in all likelihood a relatively mild migraine. Those who are prone to headaches may get this type of headache, and those who are not prone to have headaches won't.

It is certainly true that stress and tension can contribute to the onset of a headache—but what doctors used to think of as "tension headache," may not really exist. [61] (See illustration No. 8 on page 47.)

What is "exertional" headache?

Exertional headache may be brought about by straining, coughing, sneezing, stooping, or bending over. Actually, it is believed to be a type of migraine. This type of headache is not serious or dangerous, but it may last as long as

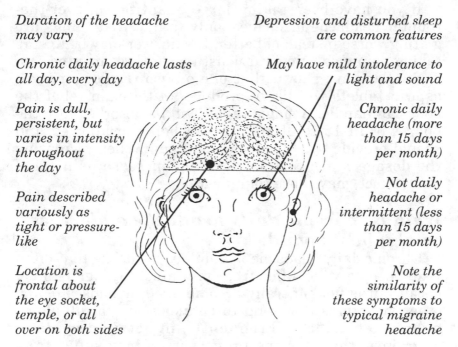

Duration of the headache
may vary

Depression and disturbed sleep
are common features

Chronic daily headache lasts
all day, every day

May have mild intolerance to
light and sound

Pain is dull,
persistent, but
varies in intensity
throughout
the day

Chronic daily
headache (more
than 15 days
per month)

Pain described
variously as
tight or pressure-
like

Not daily
headache or
intermittent (less
than 15 days
per month)

Location is
frontal about
the eye socket,
temple, or all
over on both sides

Note the
similarity of
these symptoms to
typical migraine
headache

May be aggravated by alcohol or exertion

Illustration by Lisa Price

Illustration 8. Tension-Type (So called "Tension") Headache

several hours. This type of headache is remarkably responsive to indomethacin, one of the nonsteroidal anti-inflammatory drugs (NSAIDs). [18, 21, 41, 61]

Can over-the-counter headache remedies actually make things worse?

If you are a chronic headache sufferer, you need to know that relying too heavily on any analgesic may actually make your headaches worse—and more frequent. This is the "analgesic rebound headache" that was mentioned previously. What happens is that your body and brain come to rely on analgesics for head pain relief—and, in fact, require ever larger and more frequent doses to keep the pain under control. What it boils down to, really, is that you have over medicated yourself, and your body has become conditioned to the medication.

If you have been taking large quantities of over-the-counter headache medicines, only to find that things are getting worse instead of better, the answer may be to stop taking pain medicine for at least two or three months.

Studies have shown that one or two regular strength aspirin tablets will likely produce all the pain relief the body can handle. A single tablet will be absorbed into the body within 15 to 30 minutes of being swallowed and should provide two to four hours of pain relief. Increasing the dosage much further does not increase pain relief and, in fact, may cause complications. [36, 43, 44, 58, 70]

What is "chronic daily headache and analgesic rebound?"

Chronic daily headache is a milder headache that often vexes people who suffer from migraine. "Milder" simply because it is not generally accompanied by nausea or the other symptoms that tend to go along with a full-blown migraine headache. Frequently, in between bouts of migraines, the migraine prone person may suffer from what is called "**chronic daily headache**." Chronic daily headache simply means the everyday occurrence of headache or near daily headache. Usually patients with chronic daily headache also have more severe attacks of typical migraine without aura accompanied by nausea and vomiting and other migrainous symptoms. The case of "Carol" on page 51 is an example of this problem. [36]

Then what brings about chronic daily headache? Most of the time, after eight to ten years of too-frequent analgesic use, the "in-between headaches" become more frequent—and finally take place on a daily or near daily basis. [43, 44, 58, 60] Most headache specialists feel that chronic daily headache *also* is caused by a disturbance in the brain's messengers, or neurotransmitters, such as serotonin, just as in migraine. [61] Chronic daily headache, sometimes referred to as "tension-type" headache, is frequently triggered by stress and tension, and is often the alias of "**analgesic rebound headache**." About two-thirds of patients who visit headache clinics for help suffer from a combination of migraine without aura and chronic daily headache, usually from analgesic rebound. [36]

Fully forty percent of patients who come to headache clinics suffer from chronic daily headache *alone*. Patients with migraine without aura *plus* chronic daily headache and patients with chronic daily headache alone are made up primarily of those who suffer from **analgesic rebound headache**. That is, their chronic headaches have been worsened by the too-frequent use of over-the-counter headache remedies. In a small percentage of cases—estimated at 10 to 15 percent—daily headache is not associated with overusage of pain medications or analgesics. [36] Many of these patients are victims of what is called "**new daily persistent headache**." That is, the headache simply began and never stopped. Physicians often call chronic daily headache by a variety of other names; chronic tension headache, "mixed" headache, and chronic tension/vascular headache. Unfortunately, many physicians describe any nondescript daily or near daily headache simply as "tension headache." This is almost always an inaccurate description of what is actually taking place. [36]

In one study of patients who had chronic daily headache, about eighty percent actually had what is called "**transformed migraine**." [43, 44] That is, these patients early on in their headache history had clear-cut migraine attacks; but, over the years, excessive and too-frequent use of analgesics "*transformed*" this type headache into a daily headache. Thus, the difference between "new daily persistent headache" and "transformed migraine" is that transformed migraine includes a history of clear-cut episodic migraine attacks, usually beginning when the victim is in his or her teens or early twenties. Gradually, the headaches become less intense but more frequent, to the point that by the time the patient reaches thirty-five or forty years of age, his or her head aches on an almost daily basis. Nine out of ten of these patients suffer from migraine without aura, and they usually report other symptoms such as nausea, and women report that their pain is worse during menstruation.

Interestingly, fully sixty percent of headache sufferers who have transformed migraine say that their head pain occurs on one side of the head or in the forehead, or temple. When the more severe migraine episodes strike, they are almost always in the same locations on the head as the low-grade chronic daily headache. **Treatment** for transformed migraine is basically the same as that for any other type of migraine; institution of low tyramine and low caffeine diet, use of preventive antimigraine medications, biofeedback training, and behavioral modification. Fortunately, seventy-five percent of patients improve on such a program. [18, 36]

In the case of analgesic rebound headache, about one-third of patients will be improved in one month simply by stopping their pain medicines. This percentage will increase to slightly over eighty percent after three months of not taking analgesics. Therefore, these medications must be discontinued completely for eight to twelve weeks for the victim of this type headache to experience maximum relief. [60] Some of the **symptoms** of analgesic rebound headache include tiredness and weakness, nausea, restlessness and irritability, memory problems, trouble concentrating, depression, and insomnia.

"Carol"

Headache History

Carol came to us at age forty-two with a history of headaches since childhood. Her headaches were usually worse during summer and better during pregnancy. About six years before visiting our clinic, Carol's headaches became more frequent and severe, requiring bed rest at times for up to six hours. She would awaken from sleep with a dull headache at least twenty times per month. The pain was often localized to her eye sockets, crown of the head, or temples. She was rarely free of headache which usually lasted for weeks at a time.

Carol complained of extreme sensitivity to light, short term memory problems, slurred speech, and confused feelings. Her headaches were described as dull and throbbing with varying severity...oftentimes interfering with daily activities. Fatigue, stress, oversleeping, certain foods, alcohol, chewing, stooping, and bright sunlight would often trigger or worsen headaches.

Previous Treatment

Carol's physician prescribed Inderal® which caused depression and lethargy. She occasionally received Demerol® injections. Orudis® and Anaprox® helped for a while, but the headaches only returned.

My Diagnosis

Chronic Migraine Without Aura and Chronic Daily Headache.

Effective Treatment

Carol was placed on a diet free from foods known to trigger her headaches. Verapamil was prescribed to prevent headache, plus the tricyclic desipramine and Orudis®. For severe headaches, Phenergan® and Indocin® by suppository were prescribed.

Progress

Two months later, Carol said, "I feel great, like my old self again." She continued to do well with ongoing pain management through medication as needed.

Which medications can be involved in bringing on analgesic rebound headache?

Aspirin or Tylenol® with or without caffeine or codeine, such as Fiorinal® or Fioricet®, regular aspirin, Tylenol® with synthetic codeine preparations, ergotamine tartrate, propoxyphene or Darvon®, and nasal decongestants with antihistamines. The dosage and length of time it takes to bring about analgesic rebound headache has not been determined, but it appears that as few as two Fiorinals® or Fioricets® taken every day may bring about this syndrome. We also know that patients who take these drugs for arthritis rather than for headache, do not develop analgesic rebound. No one drug seems to be worse than any other, although nonsteroidal anti-inflammatory drugs do not seem to produce this syndrome (with the possible exception of ibuprofen).

The primary treatment for analgesic rebound headache is simply to stop taking the drugs. However, abrupt withdrawal of medication may produce unpleasant symptoms including severe headache with nausea, abdominal cramping and diarrhea, and restlessness and mental anguish. This is especially true with Fiorinal® and Fioricet®, because these medications include a barbiturate. These symptoms may persist for up to seven days, but after that, the patient should notice improvement in his condition. Although simply stopping the medication produces marked improvement in many patients, the percentage increases drastically with the addition of other prophylactic antimigraine preventive medications. Patients consistently report a decrease in headaches, along with a marked decrease in irritability, depression, and mental anguish.

Effective treatment of analgesic rebound should include the following:

1) Stop usage of the offending drugs.
2) Use of medications such as IV DHE45® to break the cycle of continuing headaches.
3) Use of prophylactic medications used to prevent migraine.
4) Behavioral modification or altered life-style and

biofeedback training as well as counseling, family therapy, and physical exercise.
5) Thorough counseling with the patient regarding the ill effects of continued use of analgesics.
6) Continuity of care by the physician and other healthcare professionals.

Even with all of these measures, including hospitalization for around-the-clock intravenous dihydroergotamine therapy, about one-third of those with persistent intractable daily headache have to be hospitalized a second time. Although the vast majority of patients improve, some 20 per cent of these patients continue to be unable to work due to persistent headache. [18, 36, 42, 44, 58, 60, 61, 64, 70, 72, 73]

The cases of Margaret and Sharon on pages 54 and 55 are typical of chronic daily headache and analgesic rebound, showing how proper treatment is so beneficial.

"Margaret"

Headache History

Margaret, age forty-eight, had experienced headaches for most of her adult life. They became increasingly worse, with almost daily stabbing, hammer-like pain in the left forehead which occasionally moved to the right side. She would awaken with throbbing, severe headaches lasting hours on end. Her pain seemed to get worse during menstruation. She also experienced extreme sensitivity to light and sound, with some blurring of her vision during headache.

Previous Treatment

A non-smoker and non-drinker, Margaret took daily doses of acetaminophen, aspirin, and caffeine (about six times a day) plus numerous over-the-counter medications, prescription drugs, anti-depressants, and beta blockers...without relief. Biofeedback was without benefit, and no food triggers were apparent.

My Diagnosis

Chronic Migraine Without Aura and Analgesic Rebound Headache.

Effective Treatment

Margaret was placed on a headache diet and slowly taken off all pain medications over the next month. She was placed on verapamil and desipramine to prevent headaches. She was also instructed to take Indocin® for breakthrough headache pain and Phenergan® for nausea, both by suppository. For less severe pain, she was given Orudis® to replace the over-the-counter pain medicines upon which she had come to rely.

Progress

After one month, Margaret was improved, having had only two headaches since last seen. Two months later, she was dramatically improved and was taking no over-the-counter pain medications. Menstrual headaches continued for which she was prescribed estrogen. According to Margaret, "I feel like a new person."

"Sharon"

Headache History

Sharon came to us in 1992 at age forty-six having had headaches most of her life which she attributed to "sinus." Headaches became more severe, and she developed daily headache during the preceding seven months. Headaches were frontal with sensitivity of the scalp, face, and eyes, with stabbing, throbbing, stinging waves of pain, intolerance to light and sound, and occasional nausea and vomiting. Sharon's headaches were sometimes unbearable. They were worse at the time of ovulation and menstruation and were sometimes worsened by stress and oversleeping. Her mother and father had migraine.

Previous tests included normal CT and MRI brain scans the year before. She had taken multiple medications including amitriptyline, verapamil, Nizoral®, Midrin®, Fioricet®, Lortab®, Darvocet®, Cafergot®, and ibuprofen. Her examination, blood pressure, EEG, and lab tests were normal.

My Diagnosis

Migraine Without Aura and Analgesic Rebound Headache.

Effective Treatment

Sharon was taken off all analgesic pain medication. Her verapamil dosage was increased, and nortriptyline and desipramine were added to her treatment program. Her headaches dramatically stopped after about six weeks. Dihydroergotamine sustained release capsules were taken at the time of her periods for further relief.

Progress

She continues to do well on this program.

What is "trigeminal neuralgia?"

Trigeminal neuralgia, also known as *tic douloureux*, is a syndrome which causes pain in the lower or upper jaw-bone area on one side of the face or jaw, sometimes involving the eye area and spreading to the forehead. The *trigeminal nerve* carries sensation from the face to the brain. Studies have shown that **trigeminal neuralgia** is usually caused by an artery which lengthens and, in doing so, presses against the *trigeminal nerve* close to where it comes out of the brain stem. This painful malady generally attacks people who are in their 60's or 70's, because lengthening of the arteries is a natural part of the aging process. Slightly more women than men are affected. Many patients have reported that the pain from this disorder feels like an electric shock, and others have compared it to the "rat-a-tat" of a machine gun.

The pain of trigeminal neuralgia is almost always triggered by some activity like brushing the teeth, chewing, talking, or exposure to a cold wind—and it often occurs after dental work has been done. Frequently, the person who has this syndrome doesn't know anything is wrong until he takes a bite of food—and then he really realizes that something is wrong. In other words—it really hurts! Also, there is usually what is referred to as a "trigger zone" that cannot be touched without causing severe pain. [1, 61] (See illustration No. 9, page 57.)

Those who suffer from trigeminal neuralgia may be dramatically helped by the anticonvulsant drugs phenytoin, valproate, and carbamazepine. When treatment with these and other drugs (such as baclofen and clonazepam) does not help, a neurosurgical operation to move the artery away from the nerve may be necessary. [1, 17, 58, 61, 65, 68] An alternative to surgery involves the insertion of a heat-producing, needle-shaped electrode through the cheek under a light anesthetic. X-rays confirm that the needle is properly positioned. This electrode is electronically heated until partial coagulation of the nerve occurs. This treatment destroys certain pain fibers in the trigeminal nerve, producing some loss of sensation of the cheek and lip, but not causing the face to droop. The results of this procedure are permanent in about 80% of the cases. [1, 2, 18, 61]

The case of "Eula" on Page 58 shows an example of trigeminal neuralgia, or tic douloureux, that was controlled by Tegretol®.

Thomas' case on page 60 illustrates a similar, and yet quite different, problem due to its location, that of glossopharyngeal neuralgia, or ninth nerve neuralgia. This rare disorder also responds well to Tegretol®. Ninth nerve neuralgia is characterized by severe pains in the region of the ear and the tonsillar region of the throat. The paroxysms of pain are similar but are triggered by swallowing or yawning.

The case of "Earl" on page 59, shows how electrocoagulation of the trigeminal nerve by needle electrode gives immediate and complete pain relief in tic douloureux.

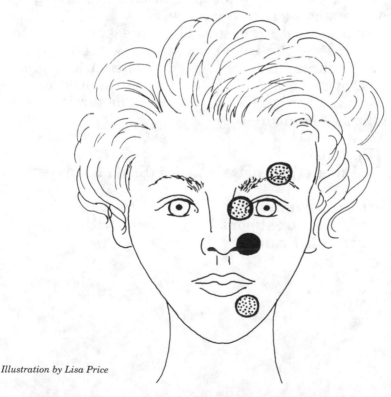

Illustration by Lisa Price

Illustration 9. Characteristic trigger zones of trigeminal neuralgia. Adapted from Raskin, N.H., Headache, *Churchill-Livingstone, Inc. New York, NY, 1988, with permission.* [61]

"Eula"

Headache History

At eighty-two, Eula was referred to our practice by her eye doctor because of recurrent pain due to tic douloureux. She was first diagnosed as having tic douloureux nine years earlier and had been treated previously with 200 milligrams per day of Tegretol® to control pain. Off Tegretol®, her pain had now returned.

When we first saw Eula, she had "tic pain" beginning in the upper lip on the left side radiating toward her left eye. She described her pains as "lightning-like," occurring repetitively for periods lasting up to fifteen minutes or longer. She also described a burning sensation in her face. The pain was sometimes triggered by chewing. She also had shingles (herpes zoster) in the same area of her face on the right side. Other than some decline in hearing, she had no other significant symptoms.

Her neurological exam and blood pressure were normal. Amazingly, the CT brain scan revealed a tumor about one inch in diameter located on the back or occipital region of the brain. This tumor was believed to be a meningioma, a benign lesion, not felt to be directly related to Eula's tic douloureux.

My Diagnosis

Tic Douloureux (Trigeminal Neuralgia) in an elderly patient.

Effective Treatment

Eula received treatment for her pain with Tegretol®, which controls her pain.

"Earl"

Headache History

Earl, a sixty-six-year-old man, consulted us while on vacation in January, 1993, because of recurrence of his tic douloureux pain over the past few weeks. He first began to have tic pain in his left jaw and tongue four years before, generally lasting about a month at a time. Earl described his pain as sharp and "electric-like," with each pain lasting about a second and occurring at ten second intervals, becoming repetitive so that they seemed to be continuous. Chewing would always precipitate the pains at the beginning of a meal. However, after a few bites he was generally able to eat without much pain for the remainder of his meal, only to have the pains return later.

Previous Treatment

His previous physician treated him with Tegretol®, which relieved his symptoms but produced unsteadiness of gait. Depakote® had been tried and did not help, and he had never taken Dilantin®. Neurological examination and blood pressure were normal.

My Diagnosis

Tic Douloureux (Trigeminal Neuralgia) of the third division of the left fifth cranial nerve.

Effective Treatment

Dilantin was tried which gave no relief at all. A neurosurgical consultation was obtained upon his return to his hometown of Boston. He was then successfully treated with electrocoagulation of the trigeminal nerve by radiofrequency needle through the skin, immediately and completely relieving Earl's pain.

"Thomas"

Headache History

Thomas came to us at age seventy-three with a fifteen year history of pain around the right ear. Each pain lasted just a few seconds at a time and would occur repeatedly for up to fifteen times per day. The cycle of pain would last three to four days and then subside for six months or longer.

Thomas described his pain as dull with an annoying sense of numbness on the right side of his face. The pain was severe enough to awaken him from sleep on occasion.

Neurological examination was normal except for blindness in his right eye from an old right eye hemorrhage. Blood tests revealed mild anemia and kidney problems. EEG was normal.

My Diagnosis

Ninth Nerve Neuralgia (Glossopharyngeal Neuralgia).

Effective Treatment

Thomas was treated with Tegretol® two tablets per day. In just two weeks, the patient's pain was completely gone...controlled by the Tegretol®.

What is TMJ?

TMJ is the more common name for temporomandibular joint dysfunction, a disorder that can be successfully treated by an oral surgeon. People who suffer from TMJ may find it painful to chew, or open their mouths wide, and they may hear clicking noises when they do so. Unfortunately, TMJ is sometimes diagnosed when the real source of head pain is a migraine. Some people have actually had "corrective" surgery, only to be disappointed when their head pain returned.

Actually, TMJ relatively rarely brings on a headache; the pain it does cause will usually be centered in the jaw or ear. When TMJ symptoms occur, surgery sometimes may be necessary. If surgery is recommended, a second opinion may be a good idea, just to make sure that temporomandibular joint syndrome is really the problem and that surgery is necessary. [18, 61]

What are increased intracranial pressure and benign intracranial hypertension?

Headache is often the only symptom of the abrupt increase of intracranial pressure that can occur due to the malfunction of a shunt used to treat hydrocephalus, especially in children. The headache itself may be related to the rate at which the spinal fluid pressure inside the head is increasing. [15]

The case of 'Linda' on page 63 shows how increased pressure within the brain and head, which is also called hydrocephalus, can produce chronic headache. Relieving this pressure by a neurosurgical shunt operation was necessary to avoid brain damage and to bring welcome relief of the patient's headaches.

Benign intracranial hypertension, also known as *pseudotumor cerebri*, is a disorder which produces symptoms very much like those associated with a brain tumor. This problem arises because there is too much spinal fluid inside the head and surrounding the brain. This can happen either because the body is making too much spinal fluid, or because the absorptive mechanism is defective.

Symptoms of this disorder include visual blurring or even complete loss of vision for seconds at a time, ringing in the ears, and headache. Frequently, patients having pseudotumor have symptoms very much like migraine, with throbbing, pounding, splitting headache, nausea, and vomiting.

On examination of the patient, the doctor may notice swelling of the optic nerve heads in the back part of the eye or retina, signifying increased pressure. Without proper treatment, permanent visual impairment can result. A first step may be a spinal puncture, through which spinal fluid pressure can be reduced to normal.

But further treatment is necessary because spinal fluid may re-form quickly, and increased pressure will return.

The disorder is treated by acetazolamide (Diamox®), cortisone derivatives, and repeated spinal punctures. Studies such as CT scanning and MRI scanning are necessary to rule out the actual presence of a tumor. [18, 61]

Many patients continue to complain of headache long after the increased spinal fluid pressure has subsided, but, fortunately, this headache will respond to the same types of medications that are used to treat migraine.

The cases of 'Laura' and 'Rhea' on pages 65 and 66 and are examples of *pseudotumor cerebri* successfully managed with Diamox® and Decadron®.

"Linda"

Headache History

Blind from birth, forty-two-year-old Linda was referred to our clinic by another physician due to her persistent headaches beginning two and a half years earlier. She had no prior history of headache, and no family members had a history of headache.

Her pain occurred in the front of her head and occasionally involved her entire head. Several times each month, severe stabbing headaches would become unbearable.

Her other physicians had performed three CT brain scans which were reported as negative. However, an MRI brain scan had revealed enlargement of the ventricles, or cavities within the brain. The MRI scan also revealed other minor brain developmental problems thought to be present since birth. Her physicians did not believe that an increased spinal fluid pressure in the head was causing her headaches. Aside from blindness, her neurological exam was unremarkable, and her EEG was normal.

Linda was hospitalized and a spinal puncture was performed. She was treated with intravenous dihydroergotamine with no improvement. Although her spinal fluid pressure was found to be normal, we felt that her MRI scan which showed *enlarged brain ventricles* indicated increased spinal fluid pressure. No tumor was found on the scan.

My Diagnosis

Hydrocephalus. In consultation with a neurosurgeon, it was believed that increased pressure within the brain was causing Linda's headaches.

Effective Treatment

A neurosurgical procedure was performed to insert a shunt, or drain, in the ventricles of the brain to relieve the pressure. The headaches decreased over the next few weeks.

Progress

Over the following three months, Linda had no headache, and a repeat CT brain scan revealed a *decrease in ventricle size*...which meant lower pressure in the brain. She continues to be headache free and has returned to work.

"Laura"

Headache History
An overweight nineteen-year-old female, Laura, had recently experienced severe headache and blurred vision. Headaches were most severe in the front and back of her head, and she described the pain as throbbing, dull or sharp, band-like, and constant both day and night. She noted ringing in her ears, and her left ear seemed to be stopped-up. Laura had taken birth control pills in the past with only occasional headaches which were relieved by Tylenol®.

The new headache was completely different, and she discontinued taking "the pill" a few days after severe headaches began. Stress, stooping over, lying down, and physical activity all made her headaches worse.

Neurological examination was normal except for swelling of the optic nerve heads in the retinas of her eyes. A CT scan of the brain and lab studies were all normal. Spinal fluid pressure was markedly increased.

Previous Treatment
A visit to an emergency room due to severe headaches resulted in her being given DHE45® (dihydroergotamine) and a narcotic, which did not relieve her headache and caused nausea and vomiting.

My Diagnosis
Pseudotumor Cerebri (False tumor of the brain).

Effective Treatment
Laura was given Diamox® and Decadron® to relieve the increased pressure of the spinal fluid. Within two days, Laura's headaches stopped dramatically .

Progress
She continued for seven months on Decadron® and Diamox® to control spinal fluid pressure. Headaches were successfully managed with verapamil and desipramine for prevention. Cafergot® and Orudis® were prescribed for occasional pain.

"Rhea"

Headache History

Twenty-three-year-old Rhea was eighteen weeks pregnant with her first child when she first experienced constant headache with blurred vision. She also complained of hearing "ocean waves" in her right ear. Rhea was referred to me by an eye specialist who found signs of swollen optic nerve heads indicating increased pressure in her head. She had stopped smoking and drinking alcohol six months previously.

Examination of Rhea confirmed the swollen optic nerve heads and increased pressure on the brain. Her blood pressure, temperature, neurological exam, EEG, and CT brain scan were all normal. Spinal puncture revealed significantly increased pressure with normal spinal fluid, chemistries and cell count.

Previous Treatment

Earlier, Rhea's physician diagnosed her as having migraine headache and panic disorder for which she was taking Tenormin®.

My Diagnosis

Pseudotumor Cerebri (False tumor of the brain) due to increased spinal fluid pressure.

Effective Treatment

Rhea was given Diamox® and Decadron® to relieve the pressure on her brain.

Progress

One week later, Rhea's spinal fluid pressure was reduced, and her headaches improved. A month after beginning treatment, her headaches were completely gone. After another month, she again noted a rushing sound in her ears indicating increased spinal fluid pressure, and her Decadron® dosage was increased. Rhea remained on Decadron® and Diamox® throughout her pregnancy to control spinal fluid pressure, relieve headache, and preserve her vision. Upon delivery of her baby, she was able to discontinue the Decadron® and Diamox® without recurrence of her headaches or her visual problems.

Why do I always seem to have a headache on Saturday morning?

It could be because you're getting too much sleep.

When you sleep past your normal "wake up" time, you may actually be adding another trigger factor. The result: a headache. It turns out that our wake-sleep cycle is also under the control of brain cells, which send messages by serotonin. Remember, this serotonin system seems to be at fault in the production of migraine. Although over-sleeping may certainly trigger a headache, it is equally true that sleep itself is often of great benefit in relieving a headache.

The best thing to do is to set your alarm at the same time every day, even on weekends and holidays. Arising at the usual time instead of sleeping late may eliminate that "Saturday-morning headache." [18, 59, 61]

Can changes in the weather affect a headache?

Yes. Changes in barometric pressure, humidity, or wind velocity can all contribute to the onset or severity of headaches.

In fact, fully half of migraine patients report that headaches can be brought on by changes in the weather. Overall, though, only about 2 per cent of all headaches are considered to be weather-related, and one study has indicated that these changes affect the severity of headache attacks, but not necessarily the frequency.

Some of the weather changes that are most frequently associated with headaches include thunderstorms, movement of a cold front into an area, excessively hot and bright weather, and winds—specifically, certain hot, dry "ill winds", such as the Santa Ana winds of Southern California, the Desert winds of Arizona, and the Zonda winds of Argentina. The day before these winds kick up, doctors in those particular areas will note a sharp increase in the number of patients complaining of migraine headaches, depression, insomnia, and general irritability.

All of these symptoms seem to be related to an increase in small air (water) ions in the air and an increase in the ratio of positive to negative ions in the atmosphere. Apparently, a physical reaction takes place in the body of the headache patient during these changes in the weather—a reaction that is demonstrated by an increase in breakdown products of the neurotransmitter serotonin in the urine of headache sufferers at such times. [61]

Isn't hypertension likely to be the cause of a headache?

Actually, the answer is no. It is somewhat rare for hypertension to be the cause of a headache—although it does happen. Actually, it is more common for the medicines used to treat hypertension to cause the onset of a headache. Those times when severe hypertension does bring about a headache, the pain is usually located in the back part of the head. Often, a headache triggered by hypertension will occur early in the morning, waking its victim from sleep. [59, 61]

I hurt my head in an accident more than a month ago. The doctor said my injury wasn't that serious—but I keep having severe headaches. What should I do about them, and should I be worried?

Not necessarily. A nagging and persistent headache often follows a bump or blow to the head, even when the original injury is not severe. In fact, a "minor" head injury may cause even longer lasting and severe problems than a head injury which results in a skull fracture or major concussion. [9] The good news, then, is that continued pain following a head injury does not necessarily mean there is anything terribly wrong. At the same time, persistent pain even after a minor head injury may be caused by a subdural hematoma—a blood clot between the brain and the coverings of the brain. (You may recall that evangelist Robert Schuller developed a life-threatening blood clot inside the skull after bumping his head on a car door.) So, it is best to have a thorough checkup to make sure everything is all right because in most cases, there are treatments that can alleviate the pain. Headaches which continue for more than two months after severe head injury are called **"chronic post-traumatic"** headaches—and, unfortunately, they are not uncommon. [1, 3, 4, 5, 9] The frequency or severity of headaches following a head injury is not an indication of the seriousness of the injury itself. The most important thing, though, is that all proper diagnostic tests be done to insure that there is no underlying danger. It is often true that a very severe case of post-traumatic headache is brought on by a minor injury. Typical migraine headaches may even be brought on or worsened by a head injury. [3, 31] If you are suffering from prolonged headache following a head injury of some sort, you may take some comfort in the knowledge that you are not alone. Far from it. In fact, it is estimated that there are three million head injuries in the United States every year, and up to half of these cause headaches that last longer than eight weeks. [5, 8, 10] Although this headache is not likely to be serious from a medical standpoint, it can have a devastating effect on family relationships, social life, and on the victim's ability to earn a living. [1]

The person who injures his head may also suffer from what is called *"post-traumatic syndrome,"* which includes symptoms such as dizziness, fatigue, insomnia, depression, irritability, and mood swings.[9] This entire group of symptoms may persist for months or even years—and may be brought about by something as common as a "minor whiplash injury." [47, 52, 54, 56, 77] Post-traumatic headache may be made worse by coughing, bending over, exertion, stress, or exposure to bright light. It may have many symptoms similar to migraine, and, in fact, head injury may bring on a person's first-ever migraine attack, or cause more severe and more frequent headaches in those who already suffer from migraine. [26, 31] In addition to suffering from headache, these patients frequently complain of increased sensitivity to sound, ringing in the ears, forgetfulness, and anxiety. This type of headache is usually treated the same way as a migraine. Other treatments may be used to relieve the pain of post-traumatic headache. The pain from less severe post-traumatic headache may sometimes be kept under control with simple analgesics, heat, muscle relaxants, biofeedback, or other means. If an examination reveals that the head pain is caused by an injury to the occipital nerve, a nerve block may provide relief (see illustration No. 10 on page 91). In other cases, treatment will be the same as that required for headaches that were not caused by injury. Most chronic post-traumatic headaches will go away on their own within four years after the injury occurs. [28] However, about fifteen to twenty percent of victims will continue to have headaches for an indefinite period—although proper treatment can bring relief for many of these people. [17, 25, 32] But, the best way to overcome this headache is to exercise caution, or, as the signs on the buses in England say, "Mind your head." It is a good idea to wear a helmet when riding a bike or motorcycle and to seek to avoid dangerous situations in general. "Jan," whose case history follows, is a fairly typical example of someone who suffers from prolonged headache following a head injury. See also the case of Jim on page 92, which illustrates pain relief by occipital nerve blocks.

"Jan"

Headache History
At age thirty-seven, Jan had only occasional minor headache until she was injured in a serious automobile collision. She suffered a cut to her forehead and bruising of her left arm.

A week after her accident, Jan developed severe, throbbing headache with nausea, vomiting, and intolerance to light and sound. Stress, oversleeping, certain foods, and alcohol seemed to trigger her headaches, causing her to go to bed for a day or two. She had occasional numbness in her hands and feet, difficulty sleeping, and a feeling of being cold. Her mother had a history of headache.

Jan's neurological exam, blood pressure, lab tests, CT brain scan, and EEG were all normal.

My Diagnosis
Migraine Without Aura...made worse by the accident.

Effective Treatment
Verapamil and amitriptyline were prescribed to prevent headache. Indocin® by suppository was given for breakthrough headaches, and Phenergan® was prescribed to control nausea. Orudis® was prescribed for less severe headaches.

Progress
One month later, Jan was improved with Orudis® for minor pain. The Indocin® for severe headaches was not necessary. Two months later, she had only one minor headache triggered by chocolate. Six months later, she experienced only occasional headache relieved by Orudis®. She was continued on verapamil and amitriptyline for headache prevention.

How does depression relate to headache?

Many patients who suffer from chronic headache are depressed. A majority of the time, this depression is caused by the aggravation of the patient's constant battle with headache. So it is the headache that brings on the depression instead of the other way around. It's easy to see why the person with chronic headache should become depressed, especially if he or she has been to numerous doctors and tried numerous treatments without finding significant relief.

Many patients with chronic daily headache and analgesic rebound headache suffer from depression. Characteristically, these people complain of insomnia or waking up too early in the morning, problems in their sex life, fatigue, and feelings of general hopelessness. Other problems that may be associated with depression include poor memory, difficulty concentrating, indecision, and feelings of guilt brought on by their inability to function normally in life. Such a person often comes to the headache specialist in desperation, saying, "You're my last hope!"

The person who suffers from depression brought on by chronic headache should remember, first of all, that his feelings are perfectly normal. He doesn't have to feel guilty about being depressed on top of everything else he's going through. And generally, with proper treatment and relief from his headache, feelings of depression will lift.

Now it could be that the headache treatment itself has brought on the depression. Beta-blockers such as Inderal® or Corgard® may do this. Other drugs, especially tranquilizers such as Valium®, may bring an underlying depression to the surface.

If you suffer from depression brought on by headache, you are certainly not alone. Generally, though, proper and effective treatment of your headache will also put an end to depression. [59, 76]

What is giant cell arteritis?

Giant cell arteritis is an important, though not so common cause of headache among the elderly, afflicting more women than men by a 60 to 40 margin. If this disorder is not treated promptly with corticosteroids, such as prednisone, visual impairment or blindness may occur in as many as 30 to 40 per cent of victims. Thus, a quick and accurate diagnosis is extremely important.

The average age of the onset of this disorder is about 70, with giant cell arteritis being extremely rare before the age of 55. The most common symptoms include headache and an aching of the limbs called polymyalgia rheumatica, pain upon chewing, weight loss, anemia, and, as has already been mentioned, blindness. The headache is most frequently described as being dull and boring, with needle-like pains occurring in addition to the head pain— which is usually worse at night or during cold weather. Tenderness of the scalp and the area over the temporal arteries is common, and this is often so painful that even activities like resting the head on a pillow or combing the hair are impossible.

Fortunately, giant cell arteritis can be quickly diagnosed by obtaining a sedimentation rate, which is almost always markedly elevated, followed by a biopsy of the temporal artery. If the diagnosis is strongly suspected, treatment with prednisone should be instituted just as soon as the sedimentation rate is obtained. The patient can then be scheduled for a biopsy to confirm the diagnosis. [6, 18, 61]

Lila's case (on the following page) is typical in that the cause of her headache was overlooked by other physicians who saw her. She responded quickly and completely to treatment with prednisone.

"Lila"

Headache History
A sixty-two-year-old female, Lila, was referred to us by her ENT (Ear, Nose and Throat) specialist because of severe frontal headache beginning nine weeks earlier. Although she had never experienced severe headache, she now had pain in the jaw and ear areas, with a sore and tender scalp, and pain when chewing.

Her headaches were described as continuous, deep and throbbing with some sharp, needle-like pains. Pain radiated from the forehead and top of the head to the bridge of the nose and left back of the neck. Noise, fatigue, and stress seemed to make her pain worse.

Initial examination by her own physician proved negative except for an elevated sedimentation rate of **47 mm**. X-rays, CT brain scan, neurological exam, and EEG were also negative. However, we found tenderness over the vessels of the scalp and in the temples. Her sedimentation rate was repeated and was found to have increased to **105 mm**.

Previous Treatment
Lila's previous physicians had given her three courses of antibiotics, nonsteroidal anti-inflammatory drugs, corticosteroids, forehead nerve blocks, and narcotics. Nothing seemed to help.

My Diagnosis
Giant Cell Arteritis based on a biopsy finding in the right temporal artery.

Effective Treatment
Lila was treated with prednisone which rapidly stopped her headaches and decreased her sedimentation rate to normal.

Progress

A maintenance dosage of prednisone provides ongoing pain management and a normal sedimentation rate.

Special Note: The risk of not treating Giant Cell Arteritis promptly with corticosteroids is blindness. Any patient over the age of fifty-five with recent onset of head pain with tenderness of the scalp should have a sedimentation rate test performed as a screen for Giant Cell Arteritis. If the sedimentation rate is elevated, treatment with steroids should begin immediately to preserve vision, and a biopsy should be scheduled. [6, 18, 61]

What is chronic carotidynia?

Chronic carotidynia, or facial migraine, is a relatively rare cause of headache. It occurs primarily among women, and may strike at almost any age, with the majority of victims being in their forties and fifties.

Most victims of this disorder complain of pain in the jaw or neck, but they may also experience severe discomfort in the region of the eye socket as well. Generally, patients who suffer from chronic carotidynia complain of continuous dull pain, along with minutes or hours of throbbing and pounding pain which may occur up to several times per week. Occasionally, the victim of this disorder may also experience sharp ice-pick-like pains. The most prominent feature of chronic carotidynia, however, is tenderness in the neck, and swelling over the prominent blood vessel in the neck, the carotid artery. The case of 'Lillie,' which follows on page 78, demonstrates chronic carotidynia with head pain responding to triamcinolone, Naprosyn®, and ergonovine.

Carotidynia is the most common cause of recurring facial pain when there is also tenderness over the carotid artery in the neck, but a sedimentation rate should be performed to rule out the possibility of giant cell arteritis. [18, 61]

"Lillie"

Headache History
Lillie, age sixty-three, had suffered from right-sided headache and soreness of her head and neck over the right carotid artery for five years prior to coming to us in late January of 1993. Lillie was referred to us by her oncologist, who had found no evidence of recurrence of breast cancer. She had been treated with Naprosyn® and Advil®, but that did not relieve the continuous head pain or the soreness in her neck, which was worse in cloudy weather. Lillie told us that her brother also suffered from headaches, and that she had some hearing loss, especially in the left ear. She had been troubled by hypertension for 18 years, for which she was taking Calan®. She was also taking eyedrops for glaucoma. She had had surgery for breast cancer and had been treated with chemotherapy in June of 1992. An examination revealed that Lillie's blood pressure was 178/90, and a neurological examination was normal except for showing the decrease in hearing she had described. She was tender over the right internal and common carotid arteries in the neck.

My Diagnosis
Chronic Carotidynia.

Effective Treatment
Nonsteroidal anti-inflammatory drugs (NSAIDS) were discontinued, and she was begun on a two-week course of triamcinolone along with ergonovine. Within a month her headache was gone, and triamcinolone was discontinued...ergonovine was continued. Two months later she continued to be improved, but reported having occasional head pain. She had discontinued her ergonovine on her own. Her Naprosyn® was restarted because of some joint pains. Ergonovine is now controlling her headaches without causing any problems with her hypertension.

What is post-spinal headache?

Post-spinal headache is severe head pain that frequently follows a spinal tap or spinal anesthesia.

This type of headache usually begins within 48 hours of the medical procedure, but it may not occur until two weeks later. About 10 to 20 per cent of patients having a spinal puncture get post-spinal headaches, with women about twice as likely as men to get them. We also know that children under the age of 14 and patients over the age of 65 are much less likely to get this headache—although we don't know why this is true.

The pain involved with this headache is usually described as dull and throbbing, and it may be accompanied by nausea, vomiting, and stiffness of the neck. Some patients complain of blurred vision or spots in front of their eyes, along with hearing loss or ringing in the ears, dizziness, and sensitivity to bright light—the same symptoms that may occur with a migraine.

Generally, this headache begins when the patient sits up or stands up—the pain often spreading throughout the entire head and neck area—and relief can be gained by lying down or applying pressure on the abdomen.

The longer the victim of post-spinal headache stands on his/her feet, the longer it will take for the pain to leave after he or she lies down.

Fortunately for those who suffer from this headache, the pain usually goes away on its own within 48 hours. However, without treatment, it may continue for weeks, or even months.

If you must undergo a spinal tap, you should make sure that your physician is using a needle with the smallest possible diameter. You should also see to it that he or she removes the needle while you are still lying flat. And then, it's a good idea to stay lying down for at least a couple of hours once the procedure is finished. Do all of these things, and you will reduce your chances of getting post-spinal headache.

What causes this headache? Most likely, it is caused by continued leakage of spinal fluid at the puncture site. Another cause of pain may be the abrupt change in spinal fluid pressure around the brain that results when the spinal canal is punctured.

A decrease in spinal fluid volume is probably responsible for symptoms of hearing loss and ringing in the ears, especially because a decrease in pressure in the inner ear also occurs. [18, 61]

One patient in our clinic complained of clicking noises in his ears, difficulty in hearing, and prolonged bouts with hiccups following placement of a shunt for hydrocephalus. In order to correct the problem, his shunt had to be replaced.

Now that we've talked about what causes the headache, the question remains, what can be done to relieve the pain?

Fortunately, it is usually a fairly easy matter to overcome post-spinal headache.

First of all, the change in spinal pressure caused by continued leakage of spinal fluid can be relieved by a simple procedure called a "blood patch." This involves removing about a tablespoon of blood from the patient's arm and injecting it into the area of the initial spinal puncture—close to, but not into the spinal canal. This usually brings an immediate end to the head pain. In fact, on most of the occasions we have used the blood patch in our clinic, the patient has been headache free almost by the time he or she has returned from the Anesthesia Department after the procedure.

But again, doing a blood patch is not often necessary with this headache, because it usually passes by itself within two days of its onset. On the other hand, there are occasions when, even after a blood patch is done, a post-spinal headache returns after a few weeks or even months—and another blood patch is required. [18, 61]

For an example of post-spinal headache successfully managed, see 'Krystal', on the following page.

"Krystal"

Headache History

A forty-year-old woman, Krystal, was first seen in our clinic with severe headache in late August, 1993. For the preceding fifteen years Krystal had had morning headache, for which she usually took Advil®. Eight days prior to being seen at our clinic, she had awakened with her usual headache and had taken 200 mg. of Advil®. About a half hour later, she took a diet capsule which contained phenylpropanolamine. Forty-five minutes after taking the diet capsule, she developed *sudden, excruciating thunderclap headache*, in the back of the head, the *worst* she had ever had. Her blood pressure then rose to more than 170/110. She was unable to work, had continued headache all over her head, and three days later was seen in the Emergency Department of a local hospital. A CT brain scan showed no bleeding, and *following a spinal puncture she developed marked increase in headache*, especially worse when sitting or standing, with nausea and vomiting. This headache was partially relieved by lying down.

When she was seen in our office, her examination was normal. However, she was quite ill and would become nauseated and have much more headache upon sitting or standing. Because she was so ill with headache, she was hospitalized as an emergency. Upon entry to the hospital, the anesthesiologist performed an *epidural blood patch*. She had almost immediate relief of her severe head pain by the time she was taken to her room after the procedure. Krystal had some mild headache which remained following the blood patch. This subsided within 48 hours with IV DHE45®. She was discharged on Prozac® once a day and Anaprox® for recurrent mild headache pain. Because she had had sudden, severe thunderclap-like headache, an *arteriogram* was performed which showed no aneurysm. The remainder of her studies were normal.

My Diagnoses
1. Chronic Daily Headache from possible analgesic rebound from ibuprofen.

2. Elevation of blood pressure from phenylpropanol-amine and the development of Post-spinal Headache after spinal puncture.

Effective Treatment
Epidural blood patch and DHE45® continuous IV therapy with maintenance headache prevention with Prozac®.

What are sinus headaches, and how do they differ from other kinds?

No matter what you might see on television commercials, *most headaches are not caused by sinus problems*. Although it is true that sinus disease affects about one out of every eight Americans, most headaches are brought about by other causes.

To understand what causes a sinus headache, you first need to understand what a sinus is. Sinuses are actually hollow, air-filled spaces in the bone of the skull, surrounding the eyes and nose. We all have four pairs of sinuses: 1) The frontals, located over the eyes; 2) the maxillary sinuses, underneath our cheeks; 3) the ethmoids, located between the eyes and the nose; and 4) the sphenoid sinuses, which lie deep in the nasal passages behind the nose. These sinus cavities connect to the nose through small passageways which may become blocked by infection or allergy.

There are three types of sinus problems. First, acute sinus infection, or sinusitis, occurs when an active inflammation involves a sinus cavity. Such an infection may bring about head or facial pain, most often in the cheeks or the forehead, although ethmoid sinusitis generally causes pain next to the nose and in the corners of the eyes. It's hard to tell, though, simply from the location of the pain, whether the problem is in relation to a sinus infection or to a migraine or cluster headache. But if the pain is accompanied by nausea, vomiting and/or sensitivity to light and sound, then you can be fairly certain that the problem is not a sinus infection. Generally, the pain of acute sinusitis will last up to a week, and may be worsened by head movement. But again, the same characteristics also apply to migraine.

The second type of sinus problem is chronic sinusitis— a condition which may last months or even years. The person who suffers from this condition may enjoy periods of good health between bouts with sinus pain, but the problem will always return. During symptomatic periods, this person will experience increased nasal congestion, pressure over the sinuses, and draining of mucus into the throat. Chronic sinusitis may also be complicated by the development of nasal polyps which block sinus draining.

A third type of sinus problem, "baro" (meaning pressure-related) sinus obstruction or blockage is caused when sinus swelling blocks the pathway to the nasal passage. In these cases, a partial vacuum is formed in the sinus cavity, resulting in negative pressure, which in turn causes discomfort over the sinuses involved. Barosinusitis may be caused by changes in the weather or atmospheric pressure (such as would be brought about by a trip to the mountains or in an airplane). To make matters more complicated, barosinusitis may actually trigger a migraine in the person who is prone to them.

Now, back to the question...how do you know if you are suffering from sinus trouble or a migraine? By means of a CT scan of the sinuses, or a direct examination using a small telescope or endoscope, the correct diagnosis can be made. Your headache specialist can determine the exact cause and treatment for your problem. He can also guide you to an ENT surgeon skilled in endoscopic surgery if that is needed.

Remember, if you have had, over a period of many years, recurring headaches involving nausea and vomiting and sensitivity to light and sound, your headache is due to migraine, and not sinusitis. [37]

What are some other causes of headache?

To our already-lengthy list of things and conditions that can cause headaches, we can add the following: benign and malignant brain tumors, tangles of abnormal blood vessels in the brain, increased spinal fluid pressure, meningitis, glaucoma, stroke and, in rare instances as previously mentioned, elevated blood pressure or hypertension. [18, 59, 61]

The case of Dennis, which follows on page 85, illustrates a case of arteriovenous malformation—or an abnormal tangle of blood vessels—which caused migraine with aura. Surgical treatment was necessary to prevent bleeding inside the brain and to relieve migraine.

"Dennis"

Headache History

At fifty-nine, Dennis consulted us with a thirty year history of headache. Headaches would not occur for a month or two...then they would occur frequently, up to twice a day. Headaches were always preceded by "lightning-like" quivering in the left side of his vision for about twenty minutes.

This was followed by pain in the right temple, in the right rear of the head, and the back of the neck. Severe throbbing headache with nausea and vomiting would become unbearable to the point that Dennis could not work.

Dennis had cardiac surgery three months earlier. He stopped smoking three packs of cigarettes per day, but continued his daily intake of two beers or cocktails. He admitted to depression, indigestion, and back pain, and he did not sleep well and felt tired.

Previous Treatment

When headache occurred, Dennis' physician prescribed two Fiorinal® tablets with codeine, and bedrest. He continued to take Cardizem® for high blood pressure. Dennis was also previously treated for duodenal ulcer, kidney stones, and had gallbladder surgery.

My Diagnosis

Initial diagnosis was Migraine With Aura (or Classical Migraine). However, a CT scan of the brain revealed a large arteriovenous malformation (AVM) in the back of the brain on the right side. He did not respond to treatment with Cafergot® and Inderal®.

Effective Treatment

Surgical removal of the arteriovenous malformation (AVM) was required. The pathologist who studied the AVM discovered that Dennis had had several instances of bleeding, making the AVM a dangerous risk of stroke. Following surgery, the patient had no further symptoms of migraine with aura and had only occasional minor headache pain relieved by Tylenol®. Some vision to his left was lost as a result of the surgical procedure.

THE PREVENTION AND TREATMENT OF HEADACHES

• •

I n our discussion of headaches, we have certainly saved the best for last. There is good news in the world of headaches, and that good news is that help is available—and available in even greater measure as more is learned about specific types of headaches, and as effective new drugs and treatments are developed.

We have already mentioned some drugs and treatments that can relieve certain types of headache pain. Now we're going to take a more in-depth look at some preventive measures and treatments.

I understand that the use of some drugs will actually prevent the occurrence of migraine headaches. Is this true?

Yes. Over the past ten years or so, many drugs have been developed which will prevent migraine. Heart and blood pressure medications—the so called beta blockers and calcium channel blockers—are very effective in this regard and are sometimes used in combination. Tricyclic antidepressants such as amitriptyline (or Elavil®) are also very effective, although there are occasional side effects such as drowsiness, weight gain, and constipation. Other drugs that have proven to be beneficial are the antiepileptic medications phenytoin (or Dilantin®) and valproate (or Depakote®). Depakote® is quite effective when it comes to headache prevention, but it may cause weight gain, some hair loss, and possibly even disturbances in liver function. [1, 13, 14, 18, 30, 33, 34, 36, 48, 51, 59, 61, 65, 69, 76, 82]

What are nerve blocks, and how do they help to eliminate headaches?

The idea behind nerve blocks is quite simple: block the transmission of pain messages along the nerve paths, and you stop the pain itself. Specifically, what you want to do is block the nerves which carry sensation from the head to the brain. Nerve blocks and local anesthetics injected into painful areas seem to interrupt the pain cycle by decreasing the number of sensory signals coming from the head routed to the brain stem. These signals seem to trigger headache by affecting the serotonin transmission system in the brain, thereby keeping the pain going. Interruption of these signals sometimes dramatically stops headaches such as migraine, as well as the pain of occipital neuralgia. In many instances, doing this brings immediate and sometimes long-lasting relief (see illustration No. 10, page 91).

There are several nerves that can be blocked in this way. For example, blocking the occipital nerve in the back part of the head with a local anesthetic in conjunction with a steroid will provide immediate relief. So will blocking the first branch of the fifth cranial nerve, which lies just above the eye. Blocking a nerve in this way may bring several days, or even weeks of relief, even to someone who normally suffers from daily or semi-daily headaches. It has also been found that a small amount of local anesthetic placed under the skin in the areas of the most intense pain in the scalp or face can also bring relief.

Nerve blocks are an exciting breakthrough that can be performed in the doctor's office. They are effective, and they do not have the side effects that may result from the use of narcotics and other antimigraine drugs such as ergotamine. As long as the nerve block is performed by a skilled physician, it is not dangerous and may be repeated as often as necessary without significant risk to the patient.[4, 61] (See illustration No. 10.)

Jim's case on page 92 shows just how effective occipital nerve blocks may be.

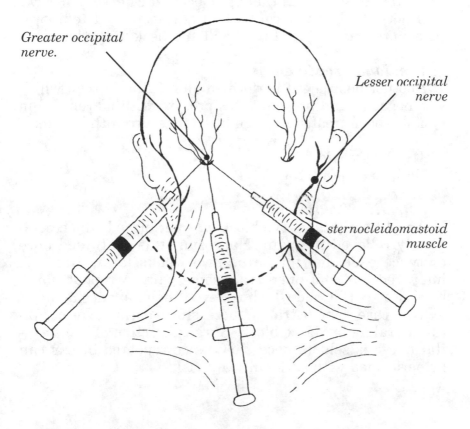

Greater occipital nerve.

Lesser occipital nerve

sternocleidomastoid muscle

Illustration by Lisa Price

Illustration 10. Technique of occipital nerve block. Adapted from Raskin, N. H., Headache, *Churchill-Livingstone, Inc., New York, NY, 1988, with permission.*[61]

"Jim"

Headache History

At fifty years of age, Jim had a three-year history of headache...occurring once or twice per day and lasting four to five hours at a time. He complained of right-sided neck pain involving his shoulder also, with dull pain in the rear right of his head.

His pain was dull, throbbing and severe...interfering with normal activities. He had no intolerance to light and sound.

His neurological exam was normal except for marked scalp tenderness over the right occipital nerve. An EEG was normal. Thermography showed decreased temperature on the right side of the head and neck in the back.

Previous Treatment

Another neurologist performed an MRI brain scan which was negative and prescribed Naprosyn® with no relief. Jim had also been treated for high blood pressure with Vasotec®.

My Diagnosis

Occipital Neuralgia.

Effective Treatment

A right occipital nerve block was performed which completely relieved the pain. Naprosyn® was continued once or twice each day for pain. Two weeks later, Jim was improved but continued with some pain. A repeat nerve block was performed which relieved the pain once again.

This case demonstrates successful treatment of occipital neuralgia by nerve block. Surgical section of the occipital nerve is seldom necessary, since repeated blocks can be performed without significant risk.

What is biofeedback?

Biofeedback is a technique used to help the victim of chronic headaches gain control over his own biological and physiological reactions to stress. Biofeedback has been demonstrated to effectively reduce or eliminate headaches in many people.

It works this way: When a human being is threatened in some way, his body gears up—either to fight or to run. This is called, quite naturally, the "fight or flight" response. When this occurs, blood flow is routed away from the intestinal tract and the skin and to the larger muscles that are going to be used in fighting or running. This, in turn, creates other changes within the body: the skin cools, the heart rate increases, and there is a tendency to perspire more. This automatic "fight or flight" response occurs in extremely stressful situations, and it frequently triggers a headache.

Biofeedback training is basically an attempt to teach the patient to learn how to block this automatic response to stressful situations, thereby preventing headaches. The biofeedback therapist does this by utilizing instruments which monitor the patient's skin temperature, perspiration, and increase in muscle contraction. All these functions can be measured easily via computer with the measurements displayed on a monitor for the patient to see. Using various relaxation techniques and other methods, the patient can actually be trained to keep his skin from cooling down, to slow the rate of his heartbeat, and—in short—to prevent the occurrence of stress-related headaches.

Biofeedback is an exciting breakthrough because, like nerve blocks, there are no side effects, no prolonged use of drugs, and—with proper training—almost anyone can become skilled in the technique. Incidentally, this method of headache control has been particularly effective among children who seem to learn it quickly and easily. They find that preventing headaches in this way can be quite a bit of fun! [11, 12]

Is there effective treatment for an acute migraine?

The drug dihydroergotamine (or DHE45®) has been proven to be an extremely effective remedy for an acute migraine, and may be given by injection, either subcutaneously (just below the skin), intramuscularly (into the muscle) or intravenously (into the vein). One or two injections an hour apart, or rarely even three injections may be necessary, depending upon the severity of the headache. The drug may be combined with a drug to prevent nausea, such as metoclopramide (or Reglan®) and prochlorperazine, (or Compazine®). [6] The new drug sumatriptan (or Imitrex®), given by subcutaneous injection, is very effective and relieves migraine within minutes.

Other drugs which may be effective in the treatment of migraine headache include ergotamine tartrate (the effective ingredient in Cafergot®) and indomethacin, both of which are more effective in suppository form than when taken by mouth. Non-narcotic analgesics such as various combinations of acetaminophen, aspirin, caffeine, and a barbiturate may also be effective—although prolonged use of analgesics may produce analgesic rebound headaches—as are various nonsteroidal anti-inflammatory anti-arthritic drugs such as naproxyn, ketoprofen, or IM ketorolac (or Toradol®). [1, 7, 18, 20, 22, 36, 50, 55, 61, 70, 72]

In short, there are many different types of drugs and drug combinations that can effectively stop acute migraine, and your doctor can help you decide which ones work best for you.

What are "trigger points" and how can they be treated to block headache pain?

Trigger points are specific areas of the body, particularly in the neck and shoulders, that may become sore or tight and thereby "trigger" headache pain. These especially painful and sensitive areas can be treated by application of heat, massage, exercise, or by the injection of a local anesthetic and steroid.

Dr. Janet Travell, who first popularized them, defined a trigger point as a location of tenderness—a sensitive area that may give rise to pain elsewhere in the body.

Trigger points may occur in muscles, skin, ligaments, or connective tissues. [79]

Trigger points are very common in adults over 25 years of age, and treatment of them can go a long way toward alleviation of headache pain.

Is there a way to prevent cluster headaches?

If you are a smoker who suffers from cluster headaches, one of the best things you can do is stop smoking. (That's really very good advice for anyone who smokes, whether or not they suffer from headaches.) Some headache specialists feel that smoke may irritate the tiny nerve fibers in the linings of the nose, and thereby increase the frequency and prolong the duration of cluster headache attacks. Sometimes a daytime nap may trigger a cluster headache, and this should also be avoided.

Also, a short course of steroids given over a period of about two weeks can bring quick control of cluster headaches. The normal course of action is to start off with larger doses of the steroid, and give increasingly smaller doses every day until stopping the treatment entirely. This two-week regimen gives time for the longer-acting maintenance medications such as verapamil and lithium carbonate to gain control of the situation and prevent cluster headaches from occurring. Ergotamine tartrate can also be used daily to prevent cluster attacks. Avoidance of alcohol, especially during cluster headache periods, and changes in diet, may also help and should be discussed with your physician. [18, 33, 34, 35, 59, 61]

Effective treatment for cluster headache

For the cluster victims who get no relief by inhaling oxygen, the two most effective measures for stopping a cluster headache attack are sumatriptan (or Imitrex®), the new serotonin "helper" drug, and dihydroergotamine (or DHE45®). Both are effective by self-injection; however, sumatriptan is much faster—often relieving headache in a few short minutes when given by subcutaneous injection by the patients themselves (personal observation). Dihydroergotamine, although effective by intramuscular or subcutaneous injection, is a bit slower and may sometimes not be effective, because some of the cluster attacks may subside by themselves in twenty to thirty minutes. It usually takes this long for DHE45® to become effective. Remember, quickness and rapidity of treatment are the watchwords in cluster headache. Since DHE45® now comes in a small glass vial, the medication must be drawn up into a syringe for use, and some time is lost by this method. DHE45® is soon to be released in a nasal spray form, not requiring injection, thus saving valuable time. [18, 23, 33, 34, 35, 40, 61] See the cases of 'Farris' and 'Roland' on pages 97 and 98 as examples of prevention of cluster and the treatment of the cluster headache attack.

An occipital nerve block, brought about by injection of a local anesthetic on the side of the head of the cluster pain, may provide relief for a week or more. Relief can also be obtained through a local anesthetic with 4 percent topical lidocaine given as a nasal drop on the side with the headache. Sometimes hospitalization for IV DHE45® around-the-clock may be necessary to bring about remission of the cluster episode.

Even though these measures can be very helpful, it is also necessary for the patient to take various preventatives or prophylactic drugs such as lithium and calcium channel blockers. [18,33,34,61,72] The cases of Farris and Roland (pages 97 and 98) show how verapamil, prednisone, oxygen, and sublingual ergotamine tartrate can bring relief from cluster headache's maddening pain.

"Farris"

Headache History

Farris, age forty-two, had a ten year history of headaches when he consulted our clinic. Recurring headaches would last from two weeks to several months only to vanish for periods up to a year and a half.

His immediate headaches began ten days earlier after a pain free period of almost three years. Headaches were always on the right side of the head beginning as a "knot" behind his right ear. Severe pain over his right eye would occur for about one hour followed by a dull ache. Whenever these headaches awakened Farris from sleep, he noticed that his right eye was extremely sensitive to light, and that his right eyelid seemed to droop.

His headaches were described as throbbing, sharp, and severe...interfering with daily activities. He was intolerant to sound, and his neck would become stiff during headache episodes. As many as three of these headaches would occur within twenty four hours, rendering him virtually incapacitated. A non-drinker, Farris smoked up to two packs of cigarettes each day, and he felt tired and depressed. His physician had performed a CT and MRI scan of the brain both of which were reported as normal.

His neurological examination, blood pressure, EEG, and lab tests were normal.

My Diagnosis

Episodic Cluster Headache.

Effective Treatment

Prednisone was begun at a relatively large dose per day, then reduced each day until the medication was gone. Verapamil was prescribed along with Cafergot® at bedtime to prevent headache pain. When cluster headaches occurred, an Ergostat® tablet was placed under the tongue, and oxygen was administered at onset of headache.

Two weeks later, Farris was free of headache. He was able to discontinue all other medications, and his cigarette smoking was reduced to half. His cluster attacks did not recur.

"Roland"

Headache History

Roland was twenty-five when he came to us with left-sided headaches which had been going on for the preceding ten days. His headaches lasted twenty minutes to two hours and were extremely painful. They began as a tight pain in the left temple with prominence of the vessels of the left temple and pain in the inner eye socket area. Headaches became throbbing and unbearable within a few minutes with runny nose, tearing, redness of the eye, and drooping of the eyelid, all on the left. Light bothered him, and if asleep in bed when headache occurred, he would awaken and get out of bed and pace. Headaches occurred up to three times a day including during the night, frequently at the same time every night. A similar bout of recurrent left-sided headaches had occurred for six weeks three years before. Five years before, he had two similar right-sided headaches.

His mother had a history of headache, but no one else in his family had headaches like his. He had smoked a pack and a half of cigarettes per day, and had consumed up to one or two cases of beer per week, but had stopped both. In the past he had duodenal ulcer. He had felt tired, nervous, and depressed.

His examination, blood pressure, and EEG were normal. Thermography showed markedly increased temperature over the left temple and eye socket characteristic of cluster headache.

Previous Treatment

Roland's other doctors diagnosed his problem as allergy. He had an operation on his nose for deviation of the nasal septum without benefit. Inderal®, amitriptyline, and various pain medications such as hydrocodone, Tylenol®, and Ergostat®, were given along with prednisone and Keflex®. Nothing helped.

My Diagnosis

Episodic Cluster Headache.

Effective Treatment
High dose prednisone on a reducing scale, verapamil, oxygen inhalation, and Ergostat® brought rapid relief and stopped the attacks.

Is there an effective treatment for shingles?

If you've never experienced shingles, consider yourself fortunate. If you have had shingles—and especially if you have them right now—you know how painful and long-lasting they can be. Shingles, known medically as **herpes zoster**, is caused by the chicken pox virus and attacks the dorsal root ganglia, or collections of nerve cells lying along the spinal cord or nerves close to the brain. Shingles features an eruption of painful blisters that may burn and itch in the area of the skin where sensation coincides with a nerve root or cranial nerve. In some cases there may be temporary paralysis of the parts of the body supplied by these nerves.

Shingles may involve the eye or ear, face, and neck. The pain can last for days, or even weeks, and once the blisters go away, the nerve pain may remain for months or longer. In short, shingles is a very nasty and painful business.

Unfortunately, there is no single drug that will quickly and effectively eliminate the pain of shingles, but there are several that will give some relief. These include the tricyclic antidepressant amitriptyline, which is especially helpful when used in combination with a phenothiazine tranquilizer. Drugs that are used to treat epilepsy—phenytoin, carbamazepine, and valproate—for example, are also helpful.[18, 22, 57, 61, 80, 81]

The eruption of shingles may indicate that the patient is physically run-down and exhausted or has a weakened immune system. Shingles is not as apt to gain a foothold in a healthy body. Therefore, an attack of shingles may indicate other physical problems that need attention.

Can changes in my diet help to prevent headaches?

Yes. Following the proper diet can greatly reduce your risk of headache. For example, if, during the course of a day, you normally drink several beverages containing caffeine—such as coffee, tea, and soft drinks—you may diminish the frequency of your headaches by cutting back to two such drinks a day. On the other hand, if you try to eliminate caffeine intake all at once, you may suffer from a headache brought on by caffeine withdrawal. A gradual cutting back is the best approach. You would also do well to limit your intake of alcoholic beverages to one per day, and total abstention is an even better idea, since alcohol is likely to be one of the most frequent triggers of a migraine. Also topping the list are chocolate and cheese. It is also a good idea to abstain from other foods containing tyramine, such as sour cream and yogurt, and to eliminate nuts and even peanut butter, and to avoid hot dogs and other foods containing nitrites, citrus fruits, and monosodium glutamate (MSG). [18, 19, 38, 46, 59, 70, 76]

The first rule of the headache diet is simply to eat three well-balanced meals a day. This will help to maintain normal glucose levels, thus, helping to prevent headaches. Headache patients who are on weight reducing diets may decrease their caloric intake, but should not skip meals altogether.

MSG is a particular problem, and although it is usually found in abundance in Chinese food, it is present in many other foods as well—especially in canned, packaged, and prepared foods. Other foods which usually contain substantial quantities of MSG include TV dinners, canned and packaged soups, chips, packaged lunch meat, salad dressing or mayonnaise, and canned or bottled sauces. If MSG is a problem for you, as it is for many headache sufferers, it's important to read labels, and to know the key words that usually mean "MSG": These include hydrolyzed vegetable protein (HVP), hydrolyzed plant protein (HPP), natural flavor, flavoring, and kombu extract. [38, 61]

What follows is a list of foods that are generally safe for headache sufferers to eat, and another list of foods that ought to be avoided:

The Headache Diet

Foods	Foods Allowed	Foods to Avoid
Beverages	Decaffeinated coffee or soda, mineral water, non-cola soft drinks, fruit juices and milk.	Coffees, teas or colas with caffeine. Drinks with aspartame (**Nutrasweet**® or **Equal**®), alcohol.
Meats	Fresh or frozen: Turkey, chicken beef, pork, lamb, fish or veal. Tuna or chicken salads.	Meats which are aged, cured, or canned. Salted or dried fish, hot dogs, pre-packaged lunch meats, and any meat that has been prepared with tenderizer or soy sauce, nuts and peanut butter.
Dairy	Two per cent or skim milk; American, cottage or cream cheese; butter, margarine, whipped cream.	Buttermilk, sour cream and other cultured dairy products. Blue, cheddar, swiss, parmesan and other types of aged cheeses.
Vegetables	Asparagus, green beans, beets, carrots, spinach, tomatoes, squash, zucchini, broccoli, corn, and lettuce.	Onions, olives, pickles, cabbage and sauerkraut. Snow peas and pea pods, broad lima, navy or pinto beans.

Foods	Foods Allowed	Foods to Avoid
Fruits	Oranges, grapefruits, tangerines, pineapples,lemons, limes—in moderation. (One-half cup per day.)	Bananas, figs, raisins, red plums, avocados.
Soups	Homemade soups and broths, if made from foods allowed.	Canned or packaged soups with yeast or MSG.
Starches	White, whole wheat or rye bread. Bagels, English muffins, French and Italian bread, crackers, most dry cereals. Irish potatoes, sweet potatoes, rice, macaroni, noodles.	Breads with yeast. Cheese crackers, and dry cereals with nuts or chocolate.
Desserts	**Jello**®, ice cream, sherbet, cakes and cookies that do not contain yeast. Yogurt (but only up to one-half cup per day).	Anything that has chocolate or aspartame.
Misc.	Salt, in moderation. Commercial salad dressings, including vinegar and oil.	Pizza, cheese sauce, macaroni and cheese, lasagna, beef stroganoff, TV dinners, soy sauce, cheese blintzes, and seasoning salt.

What is serotonin, and how are the headache drugs dihydroergotamine and sumatriptan related to it?

We've known since the 1960's that a substance known as serotonin, or 5-HT, plays a significant role in the onset of migraine. Serotonin is a chemical produced by the human body that acts as a neurotransmitter or nerve message transmitter for the brain. In other words, it carries messages from one nerve cell to another or from one nerve cell to a blood vessel. The largest concentration of serotonin in the brain is found in the brain stem.

What exactly is serotonin? It is a substance manufactured by cells in the brain and the intestinal wall. Only two per cent of the body's serotonin is found in the brain stem, but that is a vitally important two per cent, because it seems to control our sleep habits, our moods, keeps our hormones under control, and dictates how much pain we feel, or don't feel.

Research has shown that serotonin levels in the blood platelets of a person during a migraine headache are lower than those in the blood of a headache free person. When an acute attack occurs—and especially a migraine attack—the amount of serotonin in the blood decreases. What this means is that people who have inherited a tendency to have headaches regularly apparently have a disturbance in the function of nerve cells which operate by means of serotonin in the brain stem. In 85 per cent of migraine sufferers tested, increased amounts of the breakdown products of serotonin were found in their urine during a migraine.

The system of nerve cells in the brain stem which functions by means of messages transmitted by the chemical serotonin may be called the serotonin nerve cell transmission system. There is a great deal of scientific evidence that a breakdown in the proper operation of this system will result in a migraine headache.

You might think of this system as being like an automobile transmission system. When the transmission in your car begins to grind and grate, you could be headed for a breakdown. Similarly, when your serotonin system is running roughly, you may be headed for a breakdown in the form of a migraine attack. What happens is that all of the trigger mechanisms involved in setting off a migraine attack disturb the serotonin system so that it "shifts roughly." There are a number of ways the body's serotonin transmission system can be thrown off balance.

Such occurrences as a decrease in the amount of estrogen in the bloodstream at the time of menstruation may make the serotonin system function roughly, resulting in a migraine. Such chemicals found in food stuffs like tyramine, octopamine, nitrites, phenylethylamine, monosodium glutamate, and aspartame may also disturb this system and make a "breakdown" more likely. Because serotonin controls our wake-sleep cycle, it would not be difficult to see why we are more likely to get a headache if we get too much or too little sleep. Disturbances in the pattern of sleep will throw the serotonergic transmission system off balance.

Among its other functions, serotonin also constricts the larger arteries in the human brain. In fact, serotonin is the most powerful blood vessel constrictor in the brain. It also decreases pain responsiveness of the nerve cells in another part of the brain called the thalamus.

We know for certain that serotonin is involved in a headache that can be caused by administration of the tranquilizer reserpine. Reserpine brings about a decrease of serotonin in the brain, and the person who is prone to migraine will usually experience an attack within four to six hours of an intravenous injection of this drug. Fortunately, this headache can be blocked, as can other serotonin-induced headaches, by an injection of serotonin—or by two other medicines: sumatriptan and dihydroergotamine. These drugs work by mimicking or copying serotonin, thus replacing the chemical that appears to be decreased in our brain cells and blood vessels during a migraine attack. [45, 61, 66]

Sumatriptan (or Imitrex®) is absorbed easily from the intestinal tract and can be given by mouth or injection. Dihydroergotamine is not easily absorbed and must be given by injection in order to be effective, but once it has been injected, it will remain in the patient's body for about 48 hours. Either drug should do an effective job of relieving a serotonin-based headache. Sumatriptan not only relieves migraine, but the nausea that sometimes accompanies it. Dihydroergotamine may sometimes also help relieve the headache victim's nausea, but to a lesser degree than sumatriptan. [6, 7, 18, 55, 61]

Just about all medications used to prevent or relieve headaches function in some way by affecting the serotonin transmission system. Preventive headache medications seem to function by affecting different targets or receptors from those targeted by dihydroergotamine and sumatriptan. [18, 29, 36, 61, 63]

Just about the only class of medications used for headache that doesn't seem to involve the brain's serotonin system in some way are the nonsteroidal anti-inflammatory drugs (or NSAIDS). They work by blocking the formation of pain-producing substances such as prostaglandins. [18]

All of this may sound complicated and a bit confusing. But the bottom line is that over the last 25 years medical science has learned a great deal about serotonin and its role in migraine—and that knowledge has meant relief for thousands of migraine sufferers...people who once had no choice but to "grin and bear it" when headache came their way.

Should I make changes in my life-style?

There may be some areas where you need to change. For example, we mentioned before that stress may be a "trigger factor" in some types of headaches. Are you trying to do too much? Only you can answer that question— but if the most important book in your life is your Daytimer® or your Franklin® Daily Planner—then you should probably look for ways to cut back. If you don't see any possible way to cut back or avoid stress, then you may want to explore biofeedback and other relaxation techniques.

Other questions to ask yourself include, "Am I getting enough sleep?" and "Do I get enough exercise?" If you see that your daily schedule is so crowded that you are not getting enough sleep or exercise, then it is certainly time to eliminate some activities from your life.

Is it really necessary to see a doctor?

If you have persistent, recurring headache, then, yes, you should most definitely see your doctor. Too many people think the only way to deal with headaches is to grit their teeth and make aspirin and other over-the-counter remedies a steady part of their diet. We have already discussed "analgesic rebound headache," which may be brought about by prolonged use of these over-the-counter medicines. Some of these medicines work quite well for temporary relief of an occasional headache, but used regularly over long periods of time, they can actually do more harm than good.

This is one reason you should see your doctor if you suffer from chronic headache. There are two more very good reasons you should see your doctor:

1) Because there have been numerous breakthroughs in headache treatment and prevention over the past several years. It just doesn't make sense to suffer when your doctor or headache specialist can often bring you relief.

2) Because headache can be a sign of serious or even life-threatening problems that may require immediate treatment. Some people say they won't go to the doctor, because they're afraid of what he might find. That's an unfortunate attitude, because even the worst problems can often be treated if they are caught early enough. By putting off visiting your doctor, neurologist, or headache specialist, you run the risk of waiting until it's too late to do anything about the underlying problem.

Remember, though, that the source of a headache is rarely anything as ominous as a brain tumor or an impending stroke. Usually, it's something that's quite harmless, but painful—and that takes us back to point number one—that there is no reason to suffer needlessly.

"My head is killing me!"

Those words—or a variation of them—are repeated hundreds of times every day by people of every age, race, size, and life-style. Just about everyone on this planet gets a severe headache at one time or another, and millions suffer from debilitating chronic attacks that can, and often do, make their lives miserable.

Some of these people live in constant fear, never knowing when the next headache is going to ambush them. Fortunately, though, there is no need to live that way, no need to let chronic headaches ruin your life.

Final Thoughts

There is good news for headache sufferers. Incredible advances have been made in the fight against headaches. In almost every instance, freedom from headache is possible. There is an effective treatment that will work for you.

However, it's important to keep in mind that the battle against headache involves a partnership between the physician and the patient, and oftentimes even the patient's family. In other words, the headache patient must be actively involved in his treatment in order to get the best possible results.

For example, the patient must keep his physician informed, as promptly as possible, regarding any unpleasant side effects from medications that have been prescribed. He or she also must be serious about carefully following the treatment regimens and routines that are prescribed by the physician, including follow-up visits to monitor the effectiveness of drug therapy.

Over the past fifteen years, medical science has provided a number of breakthroughs in the battle against headache. But doctor and patient must work closely together to insure that the best course of treatment is followed.

During the past few years, we have seen the development and discovery of preventive medications such as beta-blockers, calcium channel blockers, tricyclic anti-depressants, antiepileptic drugs that prevent headache, and relief of headaches by medications such as indomethacin. There have been other exciting break-throughs to help relieve the individual headache attack, such as DHE45® and the startling new drug development, sumatriptan (Imitrex®), which provide an alternative to injections of narcotics. Headache specialists have even discovered that DHE45® given around-the-clock intra-venously over a few days can break the cycle of chronic daily headache that has been present for years. It had also become known that isolated migraine attacks can be transformed into chronic daily headache by the overuse of analgesics. This has drastically changed the approach to management of daily headache from analgesic rebound.

All of these exciting developments are available to you! But there is more at work here than mere medicine. Your attitude and involvement as a headache patient are so important!

For example, a positive mental attitude is a tremen-dous asset in the battle against headache. Because of this, the physician and his staff must be a source of encouragement to the patient. The body is the servant of the mind, and the evidence is becoming clearer all the time that strong, pure, and happy thoughts help to build up and renew our bodies. A positive mental attitude will ultimately express itself in good health.

Finally, it's not possible to close this book without men-tioning the power of prayer. Someone has said, "Prayer changes things," and Tennyson said, "More things are wrought by prayer than this world dreams of." Let us not forget the Biblical admonition from the Book of James that, an "effectual, fervent prayer...availeth much." [78]

This book contains a great deal of information about some of the breakthroughs that have come in the fight against migraine, cluster headache, etc. Our desire is to help you live a headache free life, and that is the aim of the information contained within these pages, and of our work at the Ford Headache Clinic. We trust that this book will be of valuable assistance as you seek to live a headache free life.

APPENDIX

∙∙

H *eadache Calendar*

Keeping a headache calendar can be a valuable tool for managing recurring headaches. For one thing, a carefully kept calendar can help the patient and his doctor identify trigger factors that might be causing migraine or other types of headaches. It can also show whether current treatments are having the desired effect, or if changes are necessary. Keep in mind, though, that in order for the calendar to be as effective as possible with regard to measuring the effectiveness of drug therapy, it must include careful monitoring of the amount of medication used each month.

Headache Calendar

MONTH _____	1	Week 1	8	Week 2	15	Week 3	22	Week 4	29
A.M. Severity									
Duration									
Medication									
Relief									
Afternoon Severity									
Duration									
Medication									
Relief									
P.M. Severity									
Duration									
Medication									
Relief									
Sleep Severity									
Duration									
Medication									
Relief									
Triggers									

Severity
1. Mild
2. Moderate
3. Incapacitating

Duration
1. Under 4 hours
2. 4-24 hours
3. 24 plus hours

Medication
1.
2.
3.

Relief
0. None
1. Slight
2. Moderate
3. Complete

Trigger
F= Foods
M= Menses
S= Stress
O= Other

112

Sample Patient Headache Calendar

MONTH _October, 1993_

		Week 1							Week 2							Week 3							Week 4									
		1	2	3	4	5	6	7	8	9	10	11	12	13	14	15	16	17	18	19	20	21	22	23	24	25	26	27	28	29	30	31
A.M.	Severity																			1	1											
	Duration																															
	Medication																															
	Relief																															
Afternoon	Severity															1		1														
	Duration																															
	Medication																															
	Relief																															
P.M.	Severity																															
	Duration																															
	Medication																															
	Relief																															
Sleep	Severity									2				2	2																	
	Duration									4				1	1																	
	Medication									3				1,2	1,2																	
	Relief													3	2																	
Triggers																M	M	M	M													

Severity
1. Mild
2. Moderate
3. Incapacitating

Duration
1. Under 4 hours
2. 4-24 hours
3. 24 plus hours

Medication
1. REGLAN
2. DHE-45
3. COMPAZINE SUPPOSITORY
4. IMITREX

Relief
0. None
1. Slight
2. Moderate
3. Complete

Trigger
F= Foods
M= Menses
S= Stress
O= Other

GLOSSARY

Acetazolamide (Diamox®) A diuretic that has proven useful in the management of pseudotumor cerebri.

Alice in Wonderland syndrome The visual aura of metamorphopsia associated with migraine, which reportedly gave rise to the characters in Lewis Carroll's classic book, *Alice's Adventures in Wonderland.* This syndrome includes illusions of altered size, shape or position of objects in the visual field, or hallucinations. It is experienced by up to 15 per cent of those who suffer from classical migraine.

Analgesic rebound headache Headache which occurs frequently, or even daily, as a result of too frequent and excessive use of painkilling medications, including over-the-counter drugs such as aspirin, Tylenol® and possibly ibuprofen.

Arteriovenous malformation (AVM) An abnormal tangle of arteries and veins occurring in the brain, which may be responsible for, or related to, migraine headache in rare instances.

Aura The visual warning of an impending migraine attack. The aura, which usually lasts about 20 minutes, includes lights flashing in front of the eyes, zig-zag lines, colors, etc.

Barosinusitis The blocking of the tiny passageways from the paranasal sinuses to the nasal cavity, which forms a small vacuum. This may occur from changes in air pressure as are brought on by such activities as mountain climbing or flying in airplanes. Even though modern aircraft are "pressurized," there are still some changes in barometric pressure which can bring on this condition.

Baclofen (Lioresal®) A muscle relaxant also useful in the treatment of trigeminal neuralgia.

Basilar migraine A severe headache which occurs most frequently in teenage girls and women under the age of 35. Along with a severe throbbing ache in the back of the head, this malady may include a number of debilitating symptoms, including dizziness, slurred speech, difficulty walking, double vision or total blindness, altered consciousness, and nausea or vomiting. The person who suffers from this headache usually craves sleep, and sleep is exactly what is needed to terminate the attack.

Benign intracranial hypertension Increased production or lack of absorption of spinal fluid, bringing on headache, visual symptoms, and swollen optic nerve heads.

Beta blockers Drugs which block the action of beta receptors. Useful in treatment of high blood pressure and in prevention of migraine.

Biofeedback A technique in which the patient learns to bring his body's involuntary responses to stress under voluntary control. Biofeedback is much more than simply a relaxation technique, and can effectively reduce the number and severity of headaches a person gets.

Brain stem The small part of the brain lying in front of the cerebellum, between the spinal cord and the cerebrum. The brain stem is a relay station responsible for controlling many of the body's vital functions. A high concentration of serotonin is found here.

Butorphanol (Stadol®) A synthetic opioid analgesic drug prepared as a nasal spray for treatment of migraine.

Cafergot® An older drug used in the treatment of migraine that mimics or enhances the action of serotonin. Cafergot contains ergotamine tartrate plus caffeine.

Calan®, Isoptin®, Verelan® Trade names for verapamil, a calcium channel blocker.

Calcium channel blockers Drugs which function by altering the entry of calcium into the body's cells. They are primarily used for treatment of high blood pressure, and are also useful in the prevention of migraine.

Carbamazepine (Tegretol®) A drug used primarily in the treatment of epilepsy, which is also quite useful in the treatment of trigeminal neuralgia.

Carotidynia Pain associated with the main artery in the neck, the carotid artery. Carotidynia includes pain in the neck, face, ear and head, along with facial pain and tenderness over the artery.

CAT scan An older term used for a CT scan. Stands for Computerized axial tomography.

Childhood migraine Migraine occurring in children prior to the onset of puberty.

Chinese restaurant syndrome A headache brought on by ingestion of monosodium glutamate (MSG), a commonly used food additive, especially in Chinese food and soy sauce. Patients who are sensitive to MSG may experience a reaction within 20 minutes of its ingestion. It usually begins with a burning sensation in the chest, which spreads to the neck, shoulders, arms and abdomen, followed by a sensation of pressure and tightness in the chest and face. Some migraine patients are especially susceptible to Chinese Restaurant Syndrome.

Chronic daily headache Headache which occurs on a daily or almost-daily basis.

Chronic paroxysmal hemicrania A relatively rare variant of cluster headache which usually occurs in women. It involves head pains which last from 5 to 45 minutes and average 12 to 15 minutes. This disorder is treated by indomethacin (or Indocin®).

Classical migraine (or migraine with aura) Migraine headaches which are preceded by various visual symptoms such as zig-zag lines and bright colored lights in front of the eyes.

Clonazepam (Klonopin®) One of the family of benzodiazepine drugs useful in the treatment of some seizure disorders and in pain problems, such as trigeminal neuralgia.

Cluster headache A severe type of recurring head pain, usually centered about the eye socket or temple. This occurs predominantly in men, with attacks generally lasting from 30 minutes to 2 hours, and averaging about 45 minutes.

Common migraine (or migraine without aura) Migraine which is not preceded by the visual warning symptoms of an aura.

Cough headache A headache brought on by coughing or exertion.

Cranial nerves Pairs of nerves that come from the lower surface of the brain and pass through openings in the skull. Cranial nerves provide sight, hearing, sense of smell and taste, sensation and movement of muscles of the face, neck, tongue, and throat and provide other vital functions. Examples: Trigeminal and Glossopharyngeal Nerves.

CT (computerized tomogram) A computer-generated X-ray of the brain or any other part of the body.

Cyproheptadine (Periactin®) A serotonin blocker used to prevent headache.

Depression A state of being down or feeling sad or hopeless. Patients with chronic pain are frequently depressed.

Desipramine (Norpramine®) One of the tricyclic antidepressants.

Dexamethasone (Decadron®) A synthetic derivative of cortisone which is useful in the treatment of acute migraine and in the management of cluster headache.

Diazepam (Valium®) A tranquilizer of the same family as Librium® and Xanax®.

Diclofenac (Voltaren®) An NSAID sometimes used in the treatment of headache.

Dihydroergotamine mesylate (DHE45®) A useful serotonin helper drug which has been around since it was first tried at the Mayo Clinic in 1945 (perhaps accounting for its name). DHE45® can stop an acute migraine attack, or administered intravenously, can stop the pain associated with analgesic rebound headache.

Divalproex (Depakote®) A drug used primarily in the treatment of epilepsy, but which is also effective in the prevention of migraine.

EEG (electroencephalogram) A recording of the electrical activity generated by the brain, just as an EKG (electrocardiogram) is a recording of the electrical activity generated by the heart.

Electrocoagulation A process by which tissues in the body, such as nerves, are broken down by heat generated electronically.

Episodic cluster headache Headache which occurs in groups or clusters, usually lasting several weeks to a few months, followed by headache free periods lasting for weeks or months. This is as opposed to chronic cluster, which persists on a daily or almost-daily basis.

Ergonovine One of the ergotamine derivatives that is useful in the prevention of migraine.

Ergotamine tartrate (Ergostat®) Ergotamine tartrate given as a tablet placed under the tongue. It is effective in the treatment of acute migraine or cluster headache.

Esgic® An analgesic which contains acetaminophen, caffeine, and a barbiturate.

Exertional headache A headache that is brought about by exertion. It usually responds favorably to treatment with Indocin®.

Fioricet® An analgesic containing acetaminophen, caffeine, and a barbiturate.

Fiorinal® An analgesic containing aspirin, caffeine, and a barbiturate.

Fiorinal #3® Fiorinal® with 30 milligrams of codeine added to it.

Fluoxetine (Prozac®) An antidepressant closely related to the tricyclic antidepressants useful in prevention of headache.

Fortification spectra A visual warning associated with the impending arrival of a migraine headache. This occurrence includes zig-zag lines which appear to be angled walls such as those that would have been built to protect a medieval town.

Giant cell arteritis A serious inflammation that begins in the arteries of the scalp, and particularly in the temples. It involves abnormally large or "giant" cells, hence the name. Untreated giant cell arteritis may lead to loss of vision.

Hemianopsia A partial loss of vision in both eyes. Homonymous hemianopsia is a condition where the loss of vision is on the same side in each eye. In other words, both eyes would experience a loss of vision to the left, or to the right.

Hemicrania continua A prolonged ache on one side of the head, which may persist for years. Hemicrania continua consists of a dull ache accompanied by jabbing, ice-pick-like pains. This type pain is specifically sensitive to Indocin®.

Hemiplegic migraine A paralysis of the arm and leg on one side of the body which sometimes occurs prior to the onset of a migraine attack. The paralysis usually lasts only 20 or 30 minutes, although it may last for hours, days, or occasionally even a few weeks.

Herpes zoster (shingles) A blister-like and very painful eruption of sores occurring in the territory of one or more sensory nerves. Shingles is caused by the same virus that causes chicken pox.

Hot dog headache A headache which occurs shortly after eating hot dogs or other cured meats. The headache is due to sensitivity to nitrates and nitrites which are used in the curing or preserving of many processed meats.

Hydrocephalus A condition in which obstruction of spinal fluid results in increased pressure within the head and brain.

Hydrocodone A synthetic codeine-like analgesic.

Hydrocodone bitartrate (Lortab®) Tylenol® plus hydrocodone, a synthetic codeine preparation (a narcotic).

Hypertension Hypertension usually refers to high blood pressure, although increased spinal fluid pressure is referred to as intracranial hypertension.

Ice cream headache A headache that stems from eating ice cream or drinking iced drinks. Ice cream headache occurs in one-third of the general population, but in about 90 per cent of those who suffer from migraines. The headache usually occurs within a few seconds after gulping cold ice cream or drink, with pain reaching its maximum strength within 25 to 60 seconds.

Ice-pick headache Sharp, jabbing head pains that occur in about 40 per cent of migraine sufferers.

Indomethacin (Indocin®) A nonsteroidal anti-inflammatory drug useful in the treatment of headache, and specifically for chronic paroxysmal hemicrania and hemicrania continua.

Intramuscular 'IM' An injection of medication into the muscle.

Intranasal The administration of drugs by sniffing them into the nasal cavity.

Intravenous 'IV' Injection of drugs or fluids into the veins.

Ketoconazole (Nizoral®) An anti-fungal drug.

Ketoprofen (Orudis®) A nonsteroidal anti-inflammatory drug used to treat headache and arthritic pain.

Ketorolac (Toradol®) An NSAID useful in the treatment of acute migraine as an injectable IM drug.

Lidocaine® **(Xylocaine)** A local anesthetic used in nerve blocks or as a nasal spray to treat cluster headache.

Lithium carbonate Medication used to prevent cluster headache. It is also used to treat bipolar manic depressive psychiatric illness.

Lumbar puncture (spinal puncture, spinal tap) Withdrawal of spinal fluid from the spinal canal in order to measure spinal fluid pressure and determine chemistries and cell count in the spinal fluid.

Meningitis Sometimes erroneously called "spinal meningitis." This disease is an infection of the actual coverings of the brain itself.

Menstrual migraine An incapacitating headache which is associated with the menstrual period.

Meperidine (Demerol®**)** A narcotic.

Mepergan® A combination of Phenergan® plus Demerol®, commonly used in emergency treatment of migraine.

Metaclopramide (Reglan®**)** An antinausea drug sometimes used to control nausea and vomiting. It is not as effective as some other antinauseants in relieving migraine.

Methysergide (Sansert®**)** A serotonin blocker which is sometimes used to prevent migraine and cluster headache. It brings about unpleasant side effects in many patients.

Midrin® An analgesic containing a mild blood vessel constrictor, a mild sedative, and acetaminophen.

Migraine equivalent A migraine aura which is not followed by a headache.

Monosodium glutamate (MSG) A food additive contained in soy sauce, Chinese foods, and many other prepared foods, which may trigger a migraine attack.

MRI (magnetic resonance imaging) A procedure which produces, by use of a giant magnet, a picture of the head, brain, or other part of the body. Similar to a CT scan or X-ray.

Naproxen (Naprosyn®**)** NSAID similar to Anaprox®.

Naproxen sodium (Anaprox®**)** A nonsteroidal anti-inflammatory drug which is useful in the treatment of headache.

Nortriptyline (Pamelor®**)** A tricyclic antidepressant similar to amitriptyline.

NSAIDS (Nonsteroidal anti-inflammatory drugs)
Drugs such as Anaprox® and Toradol®, which are primarily used for arthritis and joint and muscle pain, but which may also be used to effectively treat headache.

Occipital nerve block Blocking of the greater occipital nerve, which lies on each side of the back of the head, with a local anesthetic in combination with a steroid, in order to relieve migraine or occipital neuralgia.

Occipital neuralgia Recurrent or continuous pain in the back of the head, associated with tenderness of the occipital nerve itself.

OTC Over-the-counter drugs or pain medications.

Octopamine One of the amines occurring in citrus fruits that may trigger a migraine attack.

Orgasmic headache As the name implies, this headache is associated with sexual climax. It affects men at a ratio of four to one, is thought to be related to migraine, and can be effectively treated with Indocin® and ergotamine derivatives.

Ovulation Release of the ovum during the menstrual cycle, which may trigger headache.

Oxygen inhalation Oxygen given via mask is one of the most helpful methods of treating cluster headache.

Percodan® An analgesic narcotic drug containing oxycodone combined with aspirin. Oxycodone is similar to hydrocodone. Both are synthetic codeine-like drugs.

Phenylethylamine (PEA) A blood vessel active amine contained in chocolates, cheeses, and red wine, which may trigger headache.

Phenytoin (Dilantin®) An antiepileptic drug sometimes used to prevent migraine.

Phonophobia An intolerance to noise experienced by migraine patients.

Photophobia An intolerance to light, sometimes to the extreme, experienced by migraine patients.

Photopsia Flashes of bright light or splotches of white color, like a flashbulb going off, associated with migraine.

Post-spinal headache Headache following spinal or lumbar puncture, usually beginning within 48 hours after the procedure.

Post-traumatic headache Headache resulting from head injury—including minor injury such as whiplash. When this headache lasts longer than eight weeks, it is called chronic post-traumatic headache.

Post-traumatic syndrome A condition resulting from head injury that includes headache and other symptoms such as dizziness, ringing in the ears, memory loss or difficulty thinking, insomnia, depression, and fainting.

Prednisone Commonly used synthetic cortisone-like drug, useful in treating cluster headache.

Prochlorperazine (Compazine®) A phenothiazine antinauseant which is also a mild pain-reliever and sedative.

Promethazine (Phenergan®) An antinauseant commonly used in combination with narcotic analgesics such as Demerol®.

Propranolol (Inderal®) A beta-blocker.

Ranitidine hydrochloride (Zantac®) A histamine H-2 receptor antagonist used to treat duodenal ulcer.

Rhinorrhea Another name for a runny nose.

Scintillating scotomata Wavy lines, colors, and bright flashes or zig-zag patterns occurring as a visual warning that a migraine attack is about to occur.

Scotomata Spots in front of the eyes or loss of vision which usually occur before a migraine attack, and sometimes during the attack.

Sedimentation rate The rate at which red blood cells settle to the bottom of a test tube. Sedimentation rate indicates whether there is inflammation or infection present.

Serotonin (5-hydroxytryptamine or 5 HT) A chemical neurotransmitter, or chemical messenger in the brain. Serotonin sends messages from a nerve cell or brain cell to another nerve cell or blood vessel.

Steroid Drugs similar to cortisone and hydrocortisone which are used to reduce inflammatory response.

Sub.q. Subcutaneous injection of a drug into the fatty tissue just underneath the skin.

Subconjunctival hemorrhage A condition which sometimes occurs during a migraine attack, in which bright red blood appears in the white part of the eye between the iris and the eyelid. This condition, which generally occurs on the same side of the head as the headache, is not harmful, and will subside within two weeks.

Sumatriptan (Imitrex®) A drug that mimics the action of serotonin and is used in the treatment of acute migraine. It is administered by subcutaneous injection, and usually begins to provide relief within 15 minutes of being given.

Teichopsia ("walled vision") Temporary loss of vision in both eyes. A spot of loss of vision surrounded by bright colored lights or prisms. Teichopsia is an aura, warning of an impending migraine attack.

Temporomandibular joint dysfunction (TMJ) Pain related to dysfunction of the jaw joint. TMJ may involve difficulty in opening the mouth wide or chewing, deviation of the jaw to one side, and a clicking of the jaw or temporomandibular joint.

Tension-type headache (International Headache Society Classification) Headache lasting from 30 minutes to 7 days or longer, involving pressing, tightening, non-pulsating pain of mild to moderate intensity. Usually occurs on both sides of the head, and may include nausea, vomiting, loss of appetite, or intolerance to light and/or noise.

Thermogram/Thermography A color picture of skin temperature useful in diagnosing migraine, cluster headache, and other head pain. Thermography is the precise measurement of heat given off by the skin.

Thunderclap headache Sudden and severe onset of head pain (like an unexpected clap of thunder) which may occur as a symptom of ruptured or unruptured aneurysm.

Tic douloureux (trigeminal neuralgia) A disorder affecting the fifth cranial nerve, or the trigeminal nerve, with repeated bouts of severe pain in the forehead, upper lip and jaw, or lower lip, lasting seconds at a time, and recurring in staccato or machine-gun fashion. It is usually triggered by touching the face, by chewing, or by exposure to a cold breeze.

Triamcinolone A synthetic cortisone-like drug which is useful in the treatment of carotidynia.

Tricyclic antidepressant A variety of drugs used primarily to treat depression, but which are also useful in the prevention of migraine. Tricyclic antidepressants, such as amitriptyline and nortriptyline, block the reuptake of serotonin back into the nerve cell.

Trigger factor Any event or substance which can set off a migraine or cluster headache attack. Trigger factors may include stress and worry, exposure to bright lights, changes in weather, certain foods, etc.

Trigger point A painful or tender area in the muscle tissue just underneath the skin or around a joint. It may cause pain locally, or at another part of the body.

Tylox® An analgesic narcotic containing oxycodone and acetaminophen in combination.

Tyramine An amine contained in cheeses and other dietary products that is capable of triggering a migraine attack.

Valproate (Depakote®) An anticonvulsant, or antiepileptic drug useful in the prevention of migraine and cluster headache, and the pain of trigeminal neuralgia.

Vasotec® An antihypertensive drug used in treating high blood pressure.

Verapamil One of the calcium channel blockers used primarily for treatment of high blood pressure. Verapamil is also used to prevent migraine and cluster headache attacks.

Bibliography

1. "A Comprehensive Course in Mechanisms and Management," presented by the American Association for the Study of Headache, November 1-3, 1991.

2. Beck, D. W., Olson, J. J. and Urig, E. J. (1986): Percutaneous retrogasserian glycerol rhizotomy for treatment of trigeminal neuralgia. J Neurosurg 65:28-31.

3. Behrman, S. (1977): Migraine as a sequela of blunt head injury. Injury 9:74-76.

4. Bogduk, N. (1981): The anatomy of occipital neuralgia. Clin Exp Neurol 17:167-184.

5. Brenner, C., Friedman, A.P., Merritt, H.H., Denny-Brown, D.E. (1944): Post-traumatic headache. J Neurosurg 1:379-391.

6. Callaham, M. and Raskin, N.H. (1992): Management of Acute Headache in the Emergency Department. Am Col Emerg Physicians Video CME series.

7. Callaham, M. and Raskin, N.H. (1986): A controlled study of dihydroergotamine in the treatment of acute migraine headache. Headache 26:168-171.

8. Cartlidge, N.E.F. and Shaw, D.Λ. (1981): Head Injury. W.B. Saunders, Philadelphia.

9. Caveness, W.F. (1966): Head Injury Conference Proceedings. Caveness, W.F., Walker, A.E., (Eds) Lippincott, Phila..

10. Caveness, W.F. (1977): Incidence of craniocerebral trauma in the United States, 1970-1975. Trans Am Neurol Assoc 102: 136-138.

11. Chapman, S.L. (1986): A review and clinical perspective on the use of EMG and thermal biofeedback for chronic headaches. Pain 27:1-43.

12. Cohen, M.J., McArthur, D.L. and Rickles, W.H. (1980): Comparison of four biofeedback treatments for migraine headache: physiological and headache variables. Psychosom Med 42:463-480.

13. Couch, J.R. and Hassanein, R.S. (1979): Amitriptyline in migraine prophylaxis. Arch Neurol 36:695-699.

14. Couch, J.R., Ziegler, D.K. and Hassanein R.S. (1976): Amitriptyline in the prophylaxis of migraine. Neurology 26:121-127.

15. Dahlerup, B., Gjerris, F., Harmsen, A. and Sorensen, P.S. (1985): Severe headache as the only symptom of long-standing shunt dysfunction in hydrocephalic children with normal or slit ventricles revealed by computed tomography. Childs Nerv System 1:49-52.

16. Day, J.W. and Raskin, N.H. (1986): Thunderclap headache: symptom of unruptured cerebral aneurysm. Lancet 2:1247-1248.

17. Denker, P.G. (1944): The postconcussion syndrome: prognosis and evaluation of organic factors. NY State J M 44:379-384.

18. Dalessio, D.J., Silberstein, S.D. (Eds). (1993) Wolff's Headache and other head pain, Sixth Edition. Oxford University Press.

19. Diamond, S., Dalessio, D.J. (1986): The Practicing Physician's Approach to Headache. Fourth Edition, Williams and Wilkins, Baltimore, MD, U.S.A.

20. Diamond, S. (1984): Menstrual migraine and non-steroidal anti-inflammatory agents. Headache 24:52.

21. Diamond, S. and Medina, J.L. (1979): Benign exertional headache: successful treatment with indomethacin. Headache 19:249.

22. Drugs used for headaches and neuralgias. (1986) Drug Evaluations. AMA, Chicago, IL, 169-195.

23. Freitag, F.G. and Diamond, S. (1992): Sumatriptan in the treatment of migraine and cluster headache. National Headache Foundation Newsletter. Spring, 1992.

24. Friedman, A.P., Merritt, H.H. (1945): Relationship of intracranial pressure and presence of blood in cerebrospinal fluid to occurrence of headaches in patients with injuries to head. J Nerv Ment Dis 102:1-7.

25. Glaser, M.A., Shafer, F.P. (1932): Skull and brain traumas: their sequelae: clinical review of 255 cases. JAMA 98:271-276.

26. Haas, D.C., Pineda, G.S., Lourie, H. (1975): Juvenile head trauma syndromes and their relationship to migraine. Arch Neurol 32:727-730.

27. Henderson, W.R. and Raskin, N.H. (1972): "Hot-dog" headache: individual susceptibility to nitrite. Lancet 2:1162-1163.

28. Jacobson, S.A. (1969): Mechanism of the sequelae of minor craniocervical trauma. In Walker, A.E., et. al (Eds) The Late Effects of Head Injury. Charles C. Thomas, Springfield, IL, 501-526.

29. Jacoby, J.H., Poulakos, J.J. and Bryce, G.F. (1978): On the central antiserotoninergic actions of cyproheptadine and methysergide. Neuropharmacology 17:299-306.

30. Johnson, E.S., Ratcliffe, D.M. and Wilkinson, M. (1985): Naproxen sodium in the treatment of migraine. Cephalalgia 5:5-10.

31. Kalenak, A., Petro, D.J., Brennan, R.W. (1978): Migraine secondary to head trauma in wrestling. Am J Sports Med 6:112-113.

32. Kelly, R. Smith, B.N. (1981): Post-traumatic syndrome: another myth discredited. J R Soc Med 74:275-277.

33. Kudrow, L. (1978): Comparative results of prednisone, methysergide, and lithium therapy in cluster headache, in Current Concepts in Migraine Research, R. Greene, ed. Raven Press, New York, 159-163.

34. Kudrow, L. (1980): Cluster Headache: Mechanisms and Management, Oxford University Press, New York.

35. Kudrow, L. (1981): Response of cluster headache attacks to oxygen inhalation. Headache 21:1-4.

36. Lance, J.W. (1993): Advances in biology and pharmacology of headache. Neurology Vol. 43, (Suppl 3).

37. Levine, H.L. (1992): Sinus and headache. National Headache Foundation Newsletter. Fall, 1992.

38. Lipton, R.B., Newman, L.C. and MacLean, H. (1992): Migraine, Beating the Odds, First Edition. Addison-Wesley Publishing Company.

39. Liveing, E. (1873): On Megrim, Sick-headache, and some Allied Disorders: A Contribution to the Pathology of Nerve-Storms. Churchill, London.

40. Mather, P.J., Silberstein, S.D., Schulman, E.A., et al. (1991): The treatment of cluster headache with repetitive intravenous dihydroergotamine. Headache 31:525-532.

41. Mathew, N.T. (1981): Indomethacin responsive headache syndromes. Headache 21:147-150.

42. Mathew, N.T. (1981): Prophylaxis of migraine and mixed headache. A randomized controlled study. Headache 21:105-109.

43. Mathew, N.T., Stubits, E. and Nigam, M.P. (1982): Transformation of episodic migraine into daily headache: analysis of factors. Headache 22:66-68.

44. Mathew, N.T., Reuveni, U. and Perez, F. (1987): Transformed or evolutive migraine. Headache 27:102-106.

45. McCarthy, B.G., and Peroutka, S.J. (1989): Comparative neuropharmacology of dihydroergotamine and sumatriptan (GR 43175). Headache 29:420-422.

46. Medina, J.L. and Diamond, S. (1978): The role of diet in migraine. Headache 18:31-34.

47. Merritt, H.H., Friedman, A.P., Brenner, C. (1944): Headache and post-traumatic syndrome; clinical and experimental study. Tr Am Neurol A 70:56-60.

48. Meyer, J.S. (1985): Calcium channel blockers in the prophylactic treatment of vascular headache. Ann Intern Med 102:395-397.

49. Miller, H. (1961): Accident Neurosis. Br Med J 1:919-925; 992-998.

50. Nestvold, K. (1986): Naproxen and naproxen sodium in acute migraine. Cephalalgia 6 (Suppl 4):81-84.

51. Olerud, B., Gustavsson, C.L., and Furberg, B. (1986): Nadolol and propranolol in migraine management. Headache 26:490-493.

52. Oppenheimer, D.R. (1968): Microscopic lesions in the brain following head injury. J Neurol Neurosurg Psychiatry 31:299-306.

53. Peatfield, R.C., Glover, V., Littlewood, J.T., Sandler, M., Clifford, R.F. (1984): The prevalence of diet-induced migraine. Cephalalgia 4:179-183.

54. Povishock, J.T., Becker, D.P., Cheng, C.L.Y., Vaughn, G.W. (1983): Axonal change in minor head injury. J Neuropathol Exp Neurol 42:225-242.

55. Pradalier, A., Rancurel, G., Dordain, G., et. al. (1985): Acute migraine attack therapy — comparison of naproxen sodium and an ergotamine tartrate compound. Cephalalgia 5:107-113.

56. Pudenz, R.H., Shelden, C.H. (1946): Lucite calvarium-method for direct observation of brain. J Neurosurg 3:487-505.

57. Raftery, H. (1979): The management of postherpetic pain using sodium valproate and amitriptyline. Irish Med J 72:399-401.

58. Rapoport, A.M. (1988): Analgesic rebound headache. Headache 28: 662-665.

59. Rapoport, A.M. and Sheftell, F.D. (1990): Headache Relief. Simon and Schuster, New York.

60. Rapoport, A.M., Weeks, R., Sheftell, F., et. al. (1985): Analgesic rebound headaches: theoretical and practical implications. Cephalalgia 5(Suppl 3):448-449.

61. Raskin, N.H. (1988): Headache, 2nd Edition. Churchill Livingstone, New York.

62. Raskin, N.H. (1986): Ice cream, icepick and chemical headaches. In Handbook of Clinical Neurology, Vol. 48, ed. F.C. Rose. Elsevier Science Publishing, Amsterdam, 441-448.

63. Raskin, N.H. (1981): The pharmacology of migraine. Annu Rev Pharmacol Toxicol 21:463-478.

64. Raskin, N.H. (1986): Repetitive intravenous dihydroergotamine as therapy for intractable migraine. Neurology 36:995-997.

65. Raskin, N.H. and Schwartz, R.K. (1980): Interval therapy of migraine: long-term results. Headache 20:336-340.

66. Raskin, N.H., Hosobuchi, Y., and Lamb, S.A. (1987): Headache may arise from perturbation of brain. Headache 27:416-420.

67. Raskin, N.H. and Schwartz, R.K. (1980): Icepick-like pain. Neurology 30:203-205.

68. Ratner, E.J., Person, P., Kleinman, D.J., Shklar, G. and Socransky, S. (1979): Jawbone cavities and trigeminal and atypical facial neuralgias. Oral Surg 48:3-20.

69. Rosen, J.A. (1983): Observations on the efficacy of propranolol for the prophylaxis of migraine. Ann Neurol 13:92-93.

70. Saper, J.R. (1987): Help for Headaches, A Guide to Understanding Their Causes and Finding the Best Methods of Treatment. Warner Books, Inc.

71. Selwyn, D.L. (1985): A study of coital related headaches in 32 patients. Cephalalgia 5(Suppl 3): 300-301.

72. Silberstein, S.D. (1992): Intractable headache: Inpatient and outpatient treatment strategies. Neurology Volume 42, (Suppl 2).

73. Silberstein, S.D., Schulman, E.A., and Hopkins, M.M. (1990): Repetitive intravenous DHE in the treatment of refractory headache. Headache 30:334-339.

74. Sjaastad, O. (1993): Chronic Paroxysmal Hemicrania and Similar Headaches. In Wolff's Headache, Sixth Edition. Oxford University Press.

75. Sjaastad, O. and Spierings, E.L.H. (1984): "Hemicrania continua": Another headache absolutely responsive to indomethacin. Cephalalgia 4:65-70.

76. Solomon, S., Fraccaro, S. (1991): The Headache Book: Effective treatments to prevent headaches and relieve pain. Consumer Union of United States, Inc., Yonkers, New York.

77. Taylor, A.R., Bell, T.K. (1966): Slowing of cerebral circulation after concussional head injury. Lancet 2: 178-180.

78. The Bible, Epistle of James 5:16. King James Version.

79. Travell, J.G. and Simons, D.G. (1983): Myofascial Pain and Dysfunction: The Trigger Point Manual, Williams & Wilkins, Baltimore.

80. Watson, P.N. and Evans, R.J. (1986a): Postherpetic neuralgia: a review. Arch Neurol 43:836-840.

81. Watson, P.N. and Evans, R.J. (1986b): Treatment of postherpetic neuralgia. Clin Neuropharmacol 9:533-541.

82. Weber, R.B. and Reinmuth, O.M. (1972): The treatment of migraine with propranolol. Neurology 22:366-369.

APPENDIX

INDEX

INDEX

ABOUT THE AUTHORS

Robert Grant Ford, M.D.
Dr. Ford completed his specialty training in
Neurology at the Mayo Clinic in 1964, and began
private practice in Birmingham, Alabama, that
same year. Together with his wife, Kay, they
founded Ford Headache Clinic in 1989. Dr. Ford
has board certification in Neurology and
Electroencephalography. He is a member of the
American Association for the Study of Headache
(AASH), the American Academy of Pain
Management and is a Fellow of the American
Academy of Neurology.

Kay T. Ford, R.N.
Co-founder and Administrator of Ford Headache
Clinic, Kay Ford is a graduate of Samford
University School of Nursing in Birmingham
and has nine years' clinical experience in psychi-
atric and neurological nursing.